A Daughter's Diary

JULIE HAYDEN

A Daughter's Diary

One Woman's Journey With Her Mother's Dementia

Julie Hayden

© 2011 – Julie Hayden

All rights reserved. This book is protected by the copyright laws of the United States of America. This book may not be copied or reprinted for commercial gain or profit.

ISBN: 1475032242
ISBN-13: 978-1475032246

Scripture quotations are from The Holy Bible, English Standard Version. Copyright 2001 by Crossway Bibles, a publishing ministry of Good News Publishers. Used by permission. All rights reserved.

Statistics shared were taken from the Greater Indiana Alzheimer's Association Ambassador Volunteer Training Manual 2011.

A DAUGHTER'S DIARY

JULIE HAYDEN

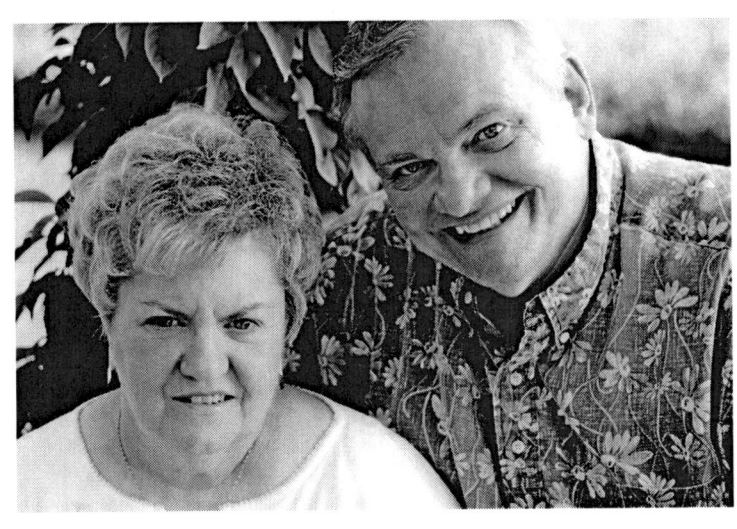

This book is dedicated to my parents,

Bill and Ruth Ann Foster

My mom was an amazing mother. She prepared me to face the hardest trial of my life – her dementia. I know she is with the Lord now and I know I will see her again. I love you, Mom!

Dad, you are an inspiration of loving to the end! You "walked her home" to heaven. You lived out your vow: for better, for worse…in sickness, and in health. Thanks for being a great example of unconditional love.

JULIE HAYDEN

CONTENTS

Special Thanks and Introduction — Xi

1. The Beginnings — 17
2. The Journal — 35
3. It's Time to Make a Change — 45
4. The Alzheimer's Unit — 55
5. The B-Wing — 65
6. The End Has Come — 73
7. Going Forward — 93
8. Lessons Learned — 95

Appendix A   Bill's Story — 109
Appendix B   Angie's Story — 111
Appendix C   Randy's Story — 115
Appendix D   Drew's Story — 117
Appendix E   The Family Song — 121

Special Thanks:

To my husband, Randy, and our children, Drew and Luke. You have been so supportive through it all. I love you.

To Dad, Michelle, Jerry, Rebekah, Angie, JJ, Madi, Macy, and Grandma. Thank you for allowing me to share our story with the world. We walked this path together and came out stronger on the other side!

To Louise. Thank you for all your hard work in editing this book. Also, thanks for your support throughout the years of this journey.

To all our faithful prayer partners, friends and ministry partners. Thank you for your faithful intercession for us while we lived this story as well as for the publishing of this book. Thank you for your gifts that made this book a reality.

To Lee Braner and Creativeleedigital for the cover photos.

To God. Thank You for Your grace every day and the strength to go on in any circumstance.

JULIE HAYDEN

Introduction

This is the story of my mother, Ruth Ann Foster. She was a great Mom and Grandma. I wish you could have known her. She was so caring and thoughtful. She sent a card for any and every occasion! She gave of herself to those she loved.

In 2005, at the age of 58, her life drastically changed. And so did mine, my father's, my sisters', as well as everyone else who was close to her. My mom was diagnosed with dementia.

Dementia will affect 1 in 8 people over the age of 65 in their lifetime. If you live to be 85, your chances of having Alzheimer's or dementia are 1 in 2. There is an epidemic about ready to break out in our nation as the baby boomers boom into these age brackets. I fear we are not ready for it!

There are no known cures or causes at this point. Medications can only help the early symptoms of this disease. They can't stop the progression; only possibly slow it down. In the end, it will be fatal.

The people diagnosed with this disease are frequently still healthy, vibrant contributors to society. Many still work and have responsibilities in their families and communities. While most common over age 65, the disease can strike as early as in the 40's.

I am part of the sandwich generation. We are "sandwiched" between caring for our children and caring for our parents. As part of this growing group, we face huge challenges of balancing the needs of our children and parents, as well as our own needs.

JULIE HAYDEN

As you read this raw account of my family's journey with dementia, I hope that you will be better equipped and prepared should you face similar issues with your family or loved ones.

"Blessed be the God and Father of our Lord Jesus Christ, the Father of mercies and God of all comfort, who comforts us in all our affliction, so that we may be able to comfort those who are in any affliction, with the comfort with which we ourselves are comforted by God."

2 Corinthians 1:3-4

JULIE HAYDEN

1 THE BEGINNINGS

Writing began June 2009

This is the story of my mother, Ruth Ann Foster. She is a beautiful woman. I wish you could know her! I want to introduce you to who she truly is!

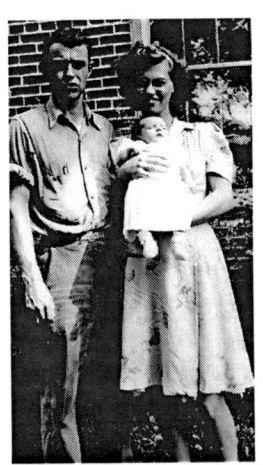

She is a baby boomer. Her father, Donald Pugsley, served in World War II. He came home and married his sweetheart, Dewala. In 1947, my mom, Ruth Ann Pugsley, was born. Dewala thought Ruth Ann was the most beautiful baby! She was so loved!!!!

A few years later, her sister, Connie, was born. They were your typical hard-working, God-fearing, middle class, small town, Midwestern family. The town had an elementary school, middle school and high school all right next to each other. My grandma worked as a cook at the school.

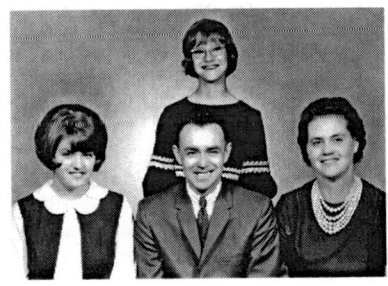

My mom sang in the choir at school. She took piano lessons. She was a cheerleader. She was very friendly and kind. During her senior year, she visited Washington DC on a class trip. She remembers the day President Kennedy was shot and could tell you what class she was in when she heard the news.

After high school graduation, she studied at a local business college. She wanted to be a secretary. She even worked for a while at a local radio station. When she would enter the broadcasting room, the DJ would say "Sunshine" had just brought them an update.

My mom met my dad on a blind date. Mom's cousin, Mary Ellen, set them up. My dad was attending a college in the next town over.

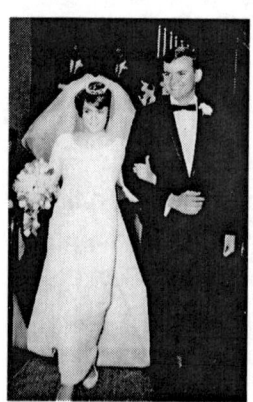

For my dad, it was love at first sight. He knew she was special, and he didn't want to let her get away. Although he was seeing another girl at the time, he never called his other girlfriend back and focused his attention only on my mom. He was smitten!

They dated for a while, and my dad knew this was the one! They got engaged, and soon, they were married! My mom was a beautiful bride!!! The date was January 7, 1967.

My dad was finishing up college. They had a little apartment near her parents. They both have told funny stories over the years about that tiny apartment and their first year together.

Soon, Michelle was born. They loved being parents – and especially having Grandma and Grandpa so close. But soon, that would all change.

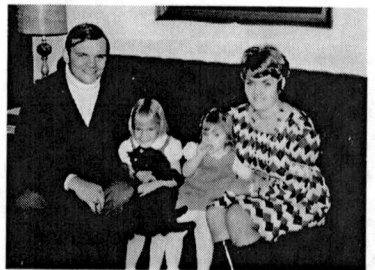

My dad discovered during his senior year that he really didn't want to be a teacher. Trying to make their way in life, my parents decided to move to the Detroit area for a few years.

Then, they moved to South Bend, Indiana. That's where I come into the picture! I was born in South

Bend in 1970. My sister, Angie, was born in 1973. Our family was complete!

I remember that living in South Bend was a lot of fun! Mom would do typing at home for extra cash. She enjoyed her work. We had the best neighbors. It was like an extended family! My mom and dad were very active in their church and made lots of friends there.

Mom sang in a ladies trio that would perform at area church services and ladies meetings. Some of my earliest memories are running through churches, playing in the nurseries while they practiced, and getting in trouble for it! ☺

My parents made life-long friends in South Bend. My parents would spend every Friday night playing cards with Doris and Denny. During the summers, we would go camping together. Doris was in the singing group with Mom. They loved being together!

On my sixth birthday, our family moved to Northwest Indiana. Dad had been out of work for a while and when a job opened up at a newspaper and printing company he took it. (Dad ended up working there until he retired.)

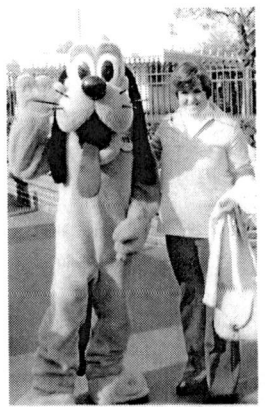

The next day we found our new church. My parents knew the minister as he had served in South Bend a few years before. We grew up in church - every Sunday morning, Sunday night and Wednesday evening, we were there! My mom sang in the choir and would help with funeral dinners. My dad was a deacon, and later, an elder. Church was a huge part of our life.

My mom and dad always wanted the best for us. When they heard about a private Christian school opening up, they sacrificed to send Angie and me there. They did not have classes for my older sister.

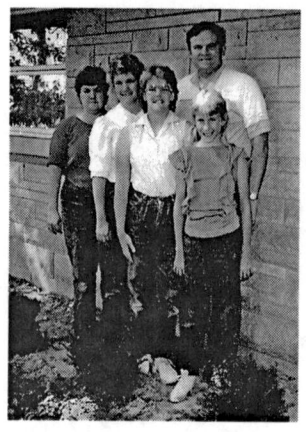

Mom ended up working at the school as an Assistant Preschool Teacher to help pay our tuition.

Mom loved working with young children! And Christmas was always fun! She would bring home the best goodies! My mom loved to decorate for every holiday, and she received many of those decorations through the students in her classes. We still have some of the handmade gifts they gave her during that time.

Mom loved Christmas! She loved to give gifts! When we were little, money was always tight, but she would really try to make it special for us. One year, she received an inheritance right before Christmas. I remember the room was so full of packages you could barely walk around in it! She loved buying for others.

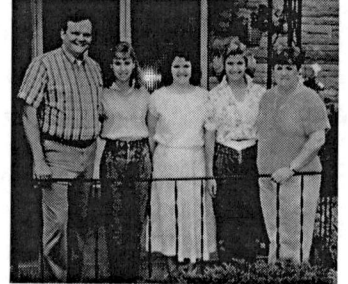

She also loved sending cards. If she heard you took your cat to the vet, she would go to Hallmark and find that special card for you! She "cared enough to send the very best!" Birthdays, anniversaries, sympathy, get well - She was always sending cards! It truly was a ministry to her.

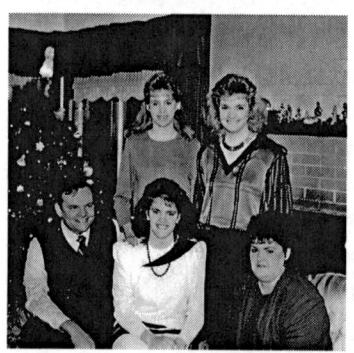

As the kids grew older, we transferred back to public school and Mom soon joined us there. She worked in the schools as a Teacher's Aide and also as a Lunchroom Cashier. She helped out where ever she could.

I think one of her favorite jobs was working at a high end dress shop. She loved fashion. She could pick out just the right outfit and accessories for anyone. She was good at it! But I think it was a job that cost her more than she made. She loved wearing the clothes too! She was a good dresser!

Mom and Dad loved to travel together. Our family vacations were always special. Mom would research and prepare a typed itinerary for our trips. My favorite trip was our trip to Washington, DC, Virginia, and Pennsylvania. We even stayed a night in a caboose motel!

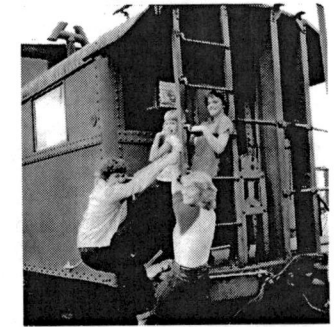

We were just a typical American family. We ate dinner at the table every night. My parents were involved in all our activities: every concert, every game, and every youth event at church. They were always there cheering us on! Mom was our personal taxi driver! She even had a license plate to prove it.

To keep it all straight, she kept a very thorough calendar. Everything was written down. She some how kept it all together. She was very organized. She called this calendar book "Her Brains". It was always an adventure when "Her Brains" came up missing!

I was the first one to go away to college. This really rocked my mom's world! It was hard to see her kids leaving the nest. During that time, she struggled with some depression and got some help from a Christian counselor during that time.

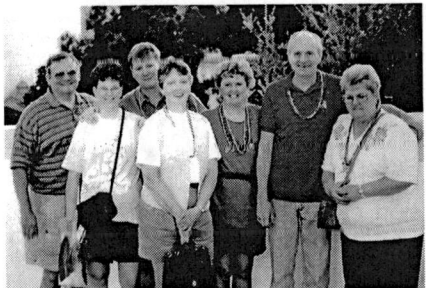

Soon she grew to love her new freedom! Dad's work was picking up. There was more disposable income. Soon they were eating out often – one of Mom's favorite things to do!!!!

During their days of being music booster parents and serving in the concession stands, they met a few couples who were doing the same thing. After all their kids had graduated, the friendships they began in the concession stand, continued with dinners and outings! They continued going each weekend to the hometown football and basketball games together. After each game, they would all go out to dinner. They began celebrating weddings and grandkids together as well!

My parents also began traveling more. They would even take some trips with their Band Booster buddies! They took trips to the Caribbean, Hawaii, Las Vegas, San Diego, and more. My parents love to travel! Their dream was to retire and travel. We even celebrated their 25th Wedding Anniversary with a cruise to the Bahamas and a stay at Disneyworld.

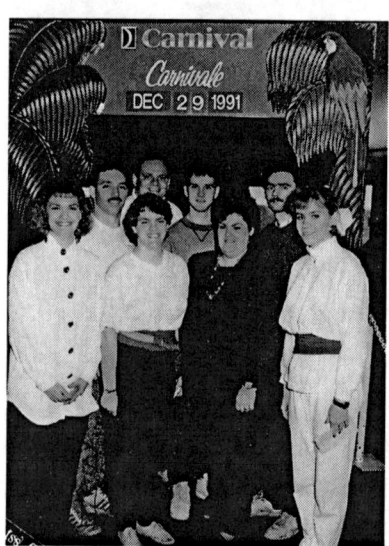

During this time, Michelle and I both got married. Michelle married her high school sweetheart, Jerry. I married Randy, whom I met on a mission trip while I was in high school. Angie was away at college where she met her man, JJ. They were married the year after they graduated.

After the clothing store where my mom worked closed, she began working for my dad's printing business. She worked in customer service and would do office work. She always enjoyed being with people and she had a blast with the ladies there!

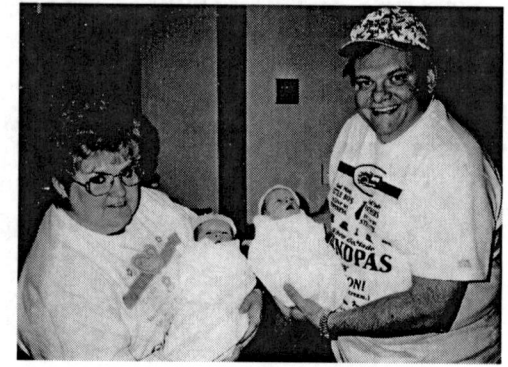

In 1995, something exciting happened in my parent's lives: they became grandparents!!! They both have said that being grandparents is even better than being parents! Mom loved being a grandma. I gave birth to twin boys, Drew and Luke in November 1995. From the first day she heard I was pregnant, she began buying gifts for the boys!

A few years later, Angie and JJ had their first girl, Madi. Mom was so happy to now have a granddaughter! She loved being able to spend time with her precious granddaughter!

Soon, Mom had two daughters pregnant at the same time! Michelle and Jerry were expecting their only child, Rebekah. Angie and JJ were expecting their second child, Macy. How fun!!!! Two babies born within a month of each other. What a great Thanksgiving we had that year celebrating the two new bundles of joy!

Being a grandma was such a huge part of Mom's life!!! She LOVED buying things for her grandchildren. Before my kids started school, she would bring a gift for them every time she came to visit. It might be a coloring book, a matchbox car, an outfit, or their favorite

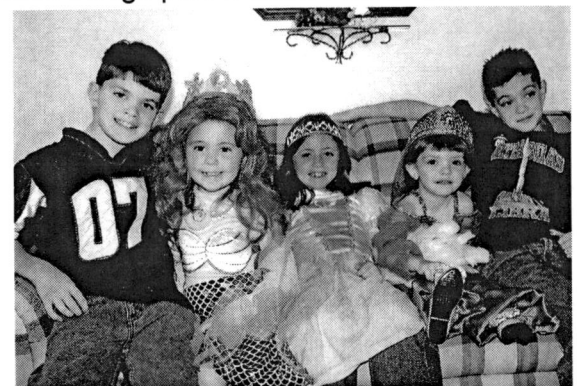

donut, but she always came bearing gifts! Her grandkids were her pride and joy!

Just like when we were kids, Mom and Dad now go to all of the grandkids' outings. They loved going to all the soccer and basketball games. They have been to gymnastic presentations, attended a myriad of school programs and music concerts, but I think their favorite was always Grandparents Day at the elementary school.

My parent's life was filled with faith, family and friends. Their life was very full! They were living the good life!

Ironically, on my mom's 50th birthday in 1997 she was diagnosed with Parkinson's disease. For eight years, she has battled with the tremors, frozen gait, and 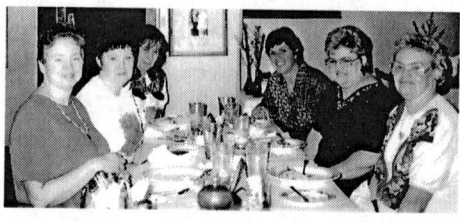 extreme movements of this disease. At first, her life changed in small ways through Parkinson's disease. In stores she would always use a shopping cart to stabilize herself. She had to give up playing piano for her church services as she would occasionally not be able to move her fingers as she needed to when playing.

When she was first diagnosed with Parkinson's disease, I remember that she shared some of her concerns with me. A family friend had suffered for years with the disease, and Mom had watched her progression from a vibrant individual, to a dependant on a family caregiver, to a resident at a nursing home. I specifically remember her sharing that her doctor mentioned that she should not lose her mental capabilities. She wasn't sure that was a great thing. She would say, "I won't be able to control my body, and I will know it!" That thought frightened her even to think about it.

Even with the physical changes, she still enjoyed a full life. She loved spending time with her five grandchildren. She still went on vacations, fishing trips to the lake, football games, and much more. She would have an occasional fall and exhibited some depression about the Parkinson's disease, but she still had many happy times with her family.

However, in 2005, at the age of 58, her life drastically changed. And so did mine, my father's, my sisters' as well as everyone else who was close to her. Mom was diagnosed with dementia.

2005

She began having irrational thoughts. At first we all just dismissed the strange happenings as effects of the Parkinson's drugs she was taking. She used to watch my children before school on mornings that I had appointments. One day while I was out of town, I had three messages from her about whether or not she should lock my door when she left. This was not like her. We always locked our doors! This should not have been an issue. The mom we knew never had trouble with such simple things.

Up until that point, she had always been organized. She loved making lists for the day with her calendar book she referred to as "Her Brains"!

Another day, she mentioned to me that while driving she had gotten turned around and temporarily didn't know where she was. She was at the main corner in our town where she had lived for over 20 years. I brushed it off as just a strange moment. Don't we all get disoriented from time to time?

Mom also began to have trouble with numbers. For years, she was the one who paid all their bills. She was in the habit of balancing her checkbook every month. She began to notice that she could not balance the bank statements any more. She was double paying some bills and forgetting others. Dad had to take back these responsibilities.

She had always been a bit of a worry wart. Now, however, she was beginning to take it to the extreme. She was paranoid about many things! She even told me that she thought my dad was having an affair – which he was not! I was not able to reason with her on it. She would say, "Yeah, you're right. But...."

Then, came Christmas Eve, 2005. She was up late and believed that there were intruders in her house. She saw many other people in her house. She saw wounded, bloody soldiers all around her living room. She thought she had been fighting with my father. She said she didn't know whether to strike out at the intruders, hurt my father, or hurt herself. While my dad was napping in the chair, Mom called the police. My dad woke up to her voice as she was hanging up the phone from calling the police. They quickly came to the house in full force! Three deep they entered the house and began questioning my father. The police soon realized that my mom was having mental issues. They calmed her down and left.

On Christmas Day, as I was preparing for the family to come over to my house, I got a call that I needed to come to their house. I could hear Mom yelling loudly in the background. Dad couldn't get her calmed down.

I rushed over there to find her crying, and my dad very upset. She was out of control again. This time, she had attacked their Christmas tree with her cane thinking it was going to hurt her. She wouldn't believe my dad that they were coming to my house to celebrate Christmas. She thought he was trying to lure her to the car to kill her. She was threatening to hurt or kill him if he tried anything, unwilling to go anywhere with him or be near him on Christmas day. She thought he was poisoning her with her medication.

I was shocked by what I was witnessing! Mom was screaming and pacing. Dad was almost in tears. How did my "peace on earth, goodwill to men" Christmas morning turn into this? Christmas was always a very special family time for the Foster's. This was not in my paradigm at all for family holidays!

After a few minutes of listening to my mom, she did let me pray with her and my father. She eventually began to calm down. I convinced her to get in my car and come to my house for Christmas dinner. Dad stayed behind for a few minutes. He put up all her medications. And he put away all the knives in the house as she was threatening to hurt him or herself. What in the world was happening!?!?!?

On December 27, 2005, my mom ended up being hospitalized for what we thought was dehydration and a medication imbalance causing the mental illness. For the few days she was in the hospital, the doctors evaluated all her medications to see what the culprit might be. It was at this time that a psychiatrist was called in for an evaluation. He was the first to mention that Mom may have dementia. Neither I, my dad, our family doctor, nor Mom's neurologist believed that to be the case. However, in three short months this prognosis would become apparent to us all.

The doctors sent her home with changes in her medications, telling us she now needed supervision until everything leveled out chemically in her body. She did improve mentally as her medications were adjusted.

She started January 2006 being at home. At first, she would stay with me or someone else during the day while my dad was at work. Little by little, she gained more freedom. Over the next few months, she began to be able to be home alone again for short periods of time and even drive. Then came the unthinkable.

March 2006

For months, Mom had been complaining of pain near her pelvic area. The doctors ran every test and x-ray possible. Mom visited her family practitioner, an urologist, and two gastroenterologists. None of these physicians could find anything wrong.

Having exhausted all other options with her doctors, we decided to try chiropractic care to see if she could get some relief from the pain. Most days, she would be fine. Yet, occasionally, she would feel a popping or sharp pain that would last for a few minutes.

As we were walking up the ramp to the chiropractor's office, Mom felt the pain again. This time is was very apparent what the problem was: her femur bone had just cracked completely in two! She stayed standing in intense pain while we waited for the ambulance. The chiropractor and her assistant came out and helped brace Mom. They were great to us!

After what seemed like a long wait, the ambulance arrived. She was put on a gurney and rushed to the nearest hospital. They ran tests and found the bone to be broken and that she needed surgery. Her surgery was scheduled for the next morning.

For the first week after her surgery, she was awake 24 hours a day! She could not be left alone in the hospital. The nurses asked us to have someone in the room with her at all times! We each took turns staying in the hospital room with Mom. Someone was there around the clock.

She spoke incessantly, making no sense what so ever, she picked at the air, tried to unbutton buttons that were not there, and carried on conversations with people and animals she thought were present in her hospital room, but were only in her mind. She used language we never heard her say before! We cried many times during this week, not knowing where our mom had gone. The lady in the bed looked like my mom, but she did not act like her at all! It was so sad!

After that week, Mom was transferred to a rehabilitation unit at another hospital. The new hospital did not require us to stay round the clock at first. It was so nice to get to sleep in my own bed!

After a short time, we learned she had injured her leg and it was broken again. We all felt she must have tried to get out of bed during the night, but no one ever told us that directly.

Following the second surgery, the hospital did require round the clock supervision. Sometimes they provided it; other times we needed to. Most of the time, I sat with Mom during the night shift since I was working from home and had the most flexible schedule. My dad was still working full-time.

Later she had one more surgery on her leg to remove infection that was settling in the wound. Each surgery was nerve racking! I remember the doctor telling us that she had lost a lot of blood during one of the surgeries.

During her time in rehab, she was supervised at all times. She was not allowed to be in her room by herself. She was back to talking more normal during the day; but at night, you never knew what you would get! This was part of the sundowners. Her dementia would be worse after the sun went down. She might not know where she was or she might be talking crazy. She just was not herself.

After two months, three surgeries, and rehab on her leg, she was physically ready to come home - yet she could not return to her house. My parents had a bi-level home with two flights of stairs. She was not able to climb stairs. We had a ranch home. My husband, Randy, built a ramp onto our house so my parents could come live with us until she could heal enough to climb stairs.

Also, Mom could no longer be left alone! We were told she had dementia along with the Parkinson's. The doctors didn't know how much she would recover mentally from all the shock, anesthetics and surgeries. My dad still worked full-time. What would we do now?

Our world was turned upside down. My parents were adjusting to their new normal in our guest room. Our family dynamics were turned upside down with everything revolving around Mom. She was like a small child, always needing attention. However, I still had a husband and two young children who needed my attention as well!

I remember going to the grocery store one night just to get away! I walked every aisle, and bought so much comfort food! I'm sure my kids loved all the ice cream bars and chocolate candy. I found peace in the grocery store! It seemed so relaxing to not be in the stress of my house for those brief two hours!

My parents lived with us for about two months before being able to return full-time to their home. My mom was glad to be going to her house. She missed her cat, Alec. Their house was transformed into a rehab center with the addition of a motorized recliner, walkers in all different varieties, raised toilet seats and bed rails.

At first, family and friends took turns watching Mom during the day while Dad worked. She knew who we were most of the time. She just could not take care of herself physically. Her mental abilities were improving slowly, but she never made a full recovery. She knew she needed the help, so she thought it was okay. She was looking forward to the day she would drive again and be alone again. She always wanted her keys to the car!

Slowly, we realized our need for help was more permanent, not temporary, and friends just could not volunteer forever. My parents had a great network of friends from their church, but there is only so much you can ask of others when it is going to be permanent.

So, my dad hired their first live-in caregiver. She did a great job of caring for my mom. She would push my mom to get better physically. She would make my mom do the things she could do for herself. Having a live-in caregiver was a really hard adjustment for my parents! Suddenly, you have someone new living with you - all the time!

December 2006

In December 2006, my mom underwent the implantation of a Deep Brain Stimulator for her Parkinson's disease. This is where they insert a device, like a pacemaker, in the brain. It helps with the impulses the brain sends. It can be adjusted to help with the symptoms associated with Parkinson's. They place the battery power pack for this device in the person's abdomen area and connect it to the brain unit with an electrode tube that is in the neck.

This device made an immediate improvement with Mom's mobility and movement. It was like a miracle! She did not need a walker or cane. She was very stable on her feet. She no longer needed help getting out of chairs or using the restroom. She was physically self-sufficient again!

However, with all the physical manifestations of the disorder nearly gone, we were left to see the tragedy of her mental condition. It was apparent just how bad mentally she had become. The physical symptoms had kept her more sedentary. Now without those restrictions, she got into a lot more trouble!

One Friday, her caregiver had to leave a few minutes before my dad got home. Previously, this had not been a problem. Mom was usually okay for a few minutes by herself. My dad was on his way home and should have been arriving within about 15 minutes. So, the caregiver left.

During those few minutes she was alone, my mom decided to wander - not just inside the house - she left their house completely. When my dad got home, he could not find her anywhere! He checked all the rooms – she was gone!

He called their friends to see if possibly someone had come to pick her up. They were planning on going to a football game that evening, but no such luck. He began looking in the yard, checking by the nearby lake, as well as searching up and down the street. When he saw the police cars down the street, his heart sank!

He went down the road to where the police cars were and found my mom. Someone saw her wandering on their busy street, stopped and got her off the road. The kind passerby waited with her until the police came. My dad was so glad that she wasn't hurt, but he was very alert to the fact that she couldn't be left alone even for a minute!

In our area, the sheriff department uses a program called "Project Lifesaver" where people at risk of wandering can have a tracking device placed in a bracelet worn on their wrist or ankle. We were able to quickly obtain one of these devices for my mom to wear in case she wandered again. Every month, a police officer would come to their house and change the batteries in the unit. This gave us great peace of mind knowing that if she did wander, she could be located!

That spring (2007), our first full-time, live-in caregiver took a different job, and we struggled with what to do. My dad was still working; my sister who lived in the area was working full-time; my other sister lived too far away. I could not handle caring for my mom full-time either with my work and family responsibilities.

The emotional drain of caring for my mom was immense. I could not emotionally and physically handle having her at my home all day. All my energy and patience would be spent by the time my family came home from work and school. I needed to be able to care for my kids too. What a hard balancing act! How do you care for two different generations with such distinct needs?

My kids tended to suffer when I had watched Mom too many days in a row. I was much less patient with them. I did not have the energy to do what they needed. Also, the confusion seemed to rub off on me. I could not make any decisions well; I felt exhausted, and did not feel like doing anything!

My husband, Randy, was great in helping me set boundaries for our family. We both were committed to helping my parents, but he could see when I was at my wits end. Because of this, he helped me set limits. I don't know what I would have done without him! We found it best for me to watch my mom for only a few hours at a time. All day, five days a week was just too emotionally draining on me. Even though I knew this was not possible, I wanted her to act like my mom, not my child.

There were other friends hired to care for my mom. My mom went to a local senior center for part of the day and would have lunch there. Then, she would have caregivers in the afternoon. Some days, I would help out for a few hours. I was always the back-up for the caregivers.

At first, Mom enjoyed the senior center. It was very nice there. They had exercise class every day. There were always musical programs and activities every day.

Overtime, and as her dementia progressed, she struggled with making friends at the senior center. Some seniors were just mean to her; they did not want to be bothered by her. She had been such a friendly person. One table of ladies welcomed her and would watch out for her. They were very kind to her.

Our local senior center wasn't equipped to provide supervision for dementia patients. As her dementia progressed, she began to need more supervision. She began to wander around the senior center's facility and grounds. The senior center's manager told us Mom could no longer attend there without assistance. We needed full-time supervision again.

Dad & I visited an adult day care center in our area. It was near his work. Adult day care provides a full range of services from supervision to bathing! This is a great resource if you are trying to keep your loved one home and you work full-time.

The problem with this adult day care was my mom would be the youngest person there by about 25 years! It was so geriatric! Everyone was in a wheelchair! We left the facility speechless after seeing the path we may have to walk in the future. We just did not want to walk it yet!

We learned about another adult day care center closer to our home. We were very relieved to learn that they had some younger clients. They also had many volunteers who dress in regular clothes who are closer to my mom's age. My mom might not feel so out of place there. This center might be a possibility in the future.

2009 (Present day as of this writing)

We were grateful when we found our second live-in caregiver. She was referred to my dad through a lady at his church. We want to keep this new caregiver for a long time. Mom goes to an adult day care some days to give the new caregiver a break. Dad takes over responsibility for Mom's care each evening when he gets home from work, plus the caregiver has every weekend off to rest and recover. We do not want to burn her out.

We are trying to put contingencies in place for Mom's future care needs. We can use the adult day care. I am willing to watch her when I can. However, we really do not want to think about the possibility of nursing home placement or even my mom's death.

Over the years, many friends from their church pitched in and did what they could. Other friends have really helped too. My parents had some friends that drew closer to them. However, some friends pulled away. I think they couldn't deal with the pain of watching what was happening.

Now, my mom has more bad days than good days. She sometimes knows me. While at other times, Mom can't quite figure out who I am. I know my mom is in there somewhere, but this is so hard for me to watch and be a part of!

This is my journal of my time with my mom from now until the end......

2 THE JOURNAL

June 30, 2009

Today, Grandma Niccum (my mom's mom) and Uncle Howard (my grandma's brother) came for a visit. Grandma Niccum lives about three hours away. It is so difficult for her to come see my mom. She loves her daughter! She is literally sick from worrying about her. Her doctor keeps telling her that she needs to stop worrying, but she says, "It doesn't matter how old she gets. She is still my daughter and you're concerned about those you love." At 84, she tells me she wishes it was her and not Ruth Ann. And I know she means it. I can not imagine what it is like to see your daughter struggling with dementia and Parkinson's disease.

Today, Mom was having an okay day. In the morning, she was somewhat content and present in the conversations. Mom seemed to enjoy our time together at their house.

While we were out to lunch, my mom just began crying for no reason. We would try to assure her everything was fine and that her mom was there, but she would just get weepy. I think she was just too tired.

I had a nice time visiting at the table with Grandma, Uncle Howard, Dad and my mom's caregiver. My mom just wasn't able to be a part of the conversation. Mom loves when Grandma comes for visits. Now, the day will pass and Mom will not remember her mother's visit. How sad....

July 6, 2009

I learned that my mom's private insurance has been cancelled by my dad's employer. With the economic downturn, the owner couldn't afford to offer health insurance any longer as an employee benefit. My dad was able to get coverage elsewhere for himself. He's healthy. My mom cannot.

Mom has qualified for disability and gets Medicare. However, now she will have no prescription coverage. Her prescriptions, just to keep her going, are over $1000 a month!!! WOW! What an eye opener to me! Dad is now looking into getting her medications from Canada as he would save almost half the price of buying them stateside. Craziness!

July 23, 2009

We really needed Mom to have a good day today! Today is the day we scheduled to go to an Elder Law Attorney to sign power of attorney papers. If Mom had a bad day and was not mentally competent, we would have to go to court for my dad to become her guardian. It would have added a lot of time, money, and stress to the situation. God was very gracious to us! Mom had a great day!

Recently, her Parkinson's doctor adjusted her medications. They turned up her deep brain stimulator and reduced her medication. It is making a world of difference!! She is able to sit still and somewhat participate in conversations.

Mom was able to understand as the lawyer explained that she needed to appoint my dad as power of attorney for when she could not make decisions for herself. She was also able to sign the house over to my dad. This is all in preparation in case she needs Medicaid or a nursing home in the future. So much to think about! I'm really glad we have an attorney who specializes in this area to walk us through all of this!

We also set up power of attorney for my dad. Oh, I hope and pray he does not pass on before my mom. I am power of attorney for him and backup for my mom. This is a huge responsibility, and I'm just beginning to realize what all it entails.

July 24, 2009

Today is another good day for Mom! She went out to dinner for ribs with her daughters and their families. What a fun time! My mom enjoyed her food. Who doesn't like great ribs?

Drew, my son, was setting next to Mom at the restaurant. He said that at one point when she had already eaten about half her food, she asked him which plate was hers. He told her and she said, "Oh good! 'Cause I'm already eating it." Drew found the timing of her question funny!

July 25, 2009

We had lunch at my house today with Mom, Dad, my sisters and their families. We had a good time just talking around the table. Dad shared about his will and the power of attorney that was put into place. Mom sat there the whole time – for about 2-3 hours! I'm just amazed at the change recently in her. I hope it is a change in the medication facilitating this, and not just the calm before a storm.

We started having these "family meetings" when Mom was hospitalized for her broken leg. These meetings have been a good tool for us to be able to all understand what is happening, come to agreement about treatments or decisions, and share our concerns. Sometimes, Grandma Niccum has been able to join us for the meetings, but not this time.

August 12, 2009

Yesterday was a really good day for Mom. She went to an adult day care facility the last two days while her caregiver was on vacation.

Mom really likes it there. She feels like she can help others who can't walk or who are worse than she is. The workers all dress in normal clothes so she doesn't fully know who is a volunteer worker and who is a patient. The staff is great, and she really fits in. It is an amazing center for people with memory issues.

I picked her up around 4:30pm. She came to my house while my dad had an appointment. She was happy!

We called my sister, Michelle, because it was her birthday. Mom was able to wish her a happy birthday, but soon after she kept losing her train of thought while on the phone. Last weekend, Michelle had had a great time with my parents. They went swimming on Saturday and then out to lunch on Sunday.

Mom said something that made me laugh. At about 5:55 pm, she said, "I need my medicine so I can stop talking." She normally takes her medicine at 6:00 pm. So I gave it to her!! The truth is that it really does help her stop talking. When the medications are wearing off, she talks all the time and she doesn't always make sense. It's just constant noise. Although I had given her the medicine, she didn't remember taking it and kept asking me for it multiple times. After about a half hour, the medicine began to work and she was again able to participate in the conversations.

We watched a few home shows on TV and then my dad arrived. I got to visit with him while he had some dinner and Mom wanted more, too. Glad I was able to have them both over for dinner. I know some day I will look back on this and wish I could do it again.

September 2, 2009

Last Friday was my Grandma Foster's 95th birthday. (Grandma Foster is my dad's mother.) We had a great time as a family celebrating this special day. It had rained most of the week and wasn't letting up, so we had the party at my house. My cousins all came. We were all together except Michelle's family who had previous plans for the night.

It just amazes me to see how well my grandma does. She seems so healthy for 95! She was part of the conversation and just enjoyed being with everyone. She can't read any more because of a degenerative eye condition, but she still is living on her own. She is very independent!

Mom seemed to have a good time at the party. She did get tired as the night wore on. She just doesn't have the stamina she used to have. In fact, she will let you know when she is ready to be done for the day!

Saturday, our clan all went out to dinner. Angie had stayed over. We went for an early dinner before my boys, Mom and Dad went to a special football game. It is nice when Mom is feeling good to get together. She was able to enjoy being at the table and not just wanting to leave.

Today, I met with the women's director at our church. Her dad just passed away after suffering with Alzheimer's. As we talked, she encouraged me to make sure I take time for me and not over commit with other involvements. She still spends time helping her mom even now that her dad has passed.

I can't forget my obligations to my family and to my parents as well. "Honor your father and mother..." keeps ringing in my head this week. Oh, Lord, help me!

September 15, 2009

This week, my mom was here on Monday. We spent the morning together while her caregiver had an appointment. We had such a nice day. Mom enjoyed blueberry pancakes for breakfast. Dad said she had wanted them recently. It is so cool how God even leads in the small things!

I did her hair. I can't believe how dry her hair gets. I have been told that it is because of her medications. She goes each week to get it done at the beauty shop, but it just doesn't hold well any more.

She always loved going to the beauty shop each week and getting her hair done for the weekend. It was her splurge after the kids were grown! One of her girlfriends picks her up each week and takes her to get her hair done and out to lunch. She knows how much it used to mean to my mom to do these things. I know it is not easy to take my mom each week, but she continues to do it. What a blessing this friend is to my mom and to our family!

We even made it to the store! As we walked through the grocery section, Mom spotted a cake mix for Red Velvet cake and cream cheese icing. She talked about wanting it, so we got it! We came home and made cupcakes. It was neat to see her enjoy them!

I have been learning to really appreciate when we have good days together. Unfortunately, that is not always the case. There are days that I get so stressed with her confusion and issues that I'm just really glad she is leaving. Oh, I hate to say that! Yet today, while she still had some confusion, overall, we had a great morning together!

November 11, 2009

Last Saturday, I spent the afternoon with my mom so Dad could take care of yard work. Mom can't be left in the house alone and the caregiver is off on weekends. She used to go outside with Dad, but now she just gets into too much trouble when he can't give her his undivided attention.

Mom and I went to the store. She seemed to be pretty good with it. It's so much easier if we have something to do rather than just sit around her house or my house. If we are just at home, she likes to get into things she is not supposed to.

While I was driving to the store, Mom said something interesting. She said, "I'm glad God had Julie come over today." I had not thought that it was God directing my steps. Yet when she said it, I realized He is guiding our steps everyday! It had not been my plan when I woke up that morning, but it just seemed like I needed to call and ask if Dad needed help.

Its funny how God's leading can be just so simple. My Mom does not make sense most of the time anymore. She didn't even realize she was talking to me, but what she said in that moment had a profound impact on me.

December 10, 2009

It has been a while since I posted. Thanksgiving hit me kind of hard. We had a great day. Mom and Dad, Grandma Foster, Aunt Suzi (my dad's sister), my sisters and their families were all able to be here for the day. That Friday, we celebrated my niece Rebekah's birthday with a bowling party. Saturday, Mom and Dad were back to watch the Indiana state football finals on our cable TV. We had a great time.

Afterwards, I was just really drained. Monday and Tuesday after having them here most of the weekend, I could do nothing! I sat in a chair, read my Bible, prayed, and read the book *Suffering in Slow Motion*. The book put into words many of my thoughts about what is happening with Mom. The story was one couples' journey through dementia and showed both the victim and the caregiver's story. It made me so sad for my mom.

I see her slipping away more and more. She is more belligerent with my dad. I've read that this type of behavior happens often with their primary caregivers. She has started having some times of quiet. More and more, there are times she is just in her own world. It seems like she is slipping away from us.

I really don't know if we will have another Thanksgiving with her. Just sad to think about it. Glad we had a nice time together this year and that we laughed a lot!

One awkward moment came when I mentioned about a friend who had received a special present from their grandma at their wedding shower. When the grandma was downsizing from her house to an assisted living facility, she had selected a special set of items from her crystal or china to be given to each grandchild. I thought it was such a neat idea and thought it would be great for my mom to select a gift for each of the grandkids that they would be given from her when they marry. Most likely Mom won't be there at that time.

My sisters and Dad thought it was great, but my grandma just looked a little unhappy about the discussion. It made me feel like I was giving away everything of Mom's even before she died. It is so hard to know what to do and what not to do. I really want her to select something for the kids so she could share in their special day. I want each of the grandkids to remember her during their wedding celebration.

Mom does not seem to be able to grasp the idea either. She told me those items are hers. She doesn't understand about leaving an inheritance piece to each grandchild. I guess the window of her selecting those items for the grandkids has passed. We will have to do it later.

I've been praying about a support group for caregivers at our church. I don't want to lead it but I see a huge need. I'm thinking about gathering a few of the daughters of dementia and doing the questions from the book *Suffering in Slow Motion*. I would really like a safe place to talk without worrying that people think I don't care about Mom when I'm just frustrated.

Dad's job also changed again. He is now home. They are still re-negotiating his contract. I wish his retirement could be something we celebrate. However, it has not come about in a good way, nor is this the retirement he hoped for. I feel so bad for him!

JULIE HAYDEN

3 IT'S TIME TO MAKE A CHANGE

March 2010

Well, a lot has changed since my last writing. Almost two weeks ago, my mom's caregiver called to let me know that things were not going well. My mom's health has declined sharply since Christmas - and my dad's patience is growing thinner. We have all seen it, but now we need to do something about it. It is time to begin looking at other options – nursing homes! I jumped into panic mode and began making plans. Now, I see God working ahead of us and making a clear path!

March 2, 2010

We visited a nursing home today for the first time. My dad doesn't want to consider nursing care yet, but we were looking at it for the future. A "just in case we need it" visit. My dad seemed to be relaxed while we were there

It started a little rough this morning. At the time we were supposed to be leaving for the nursing home, the school called saying Drew was sick and had a fever. We were able to push our meeting at the nursing home to the afternoon so I could get Drew home and resting before I had to leave.

The lady that met with us at the nursing home was very nice and made my dad feel comfortable. The facility was really nice. It seemed clean. People seemed happy. The facility offers lots of therapy options and many activities in the Alzheimer's unit. They are set up on the principles of the book, *36 Hour Day*.

One thing we learned today is that, when my mom hits the last stages of the disease, she will be moved into the regular nursing section. The residents on this unit must be able to interact with others, feed themselves, and participate in activities.

As we were leaving the nursing home, Dad mentioned he thought us girls would need to make the decision for a nursing home. He doesn't think he can do it. My dad and I decided to go for coffee to talk about it more. I encouraged him to begin the process. Just start and see where it leads. We just walk through the doors God opens – and stop if God closes them.

While we were discussing if now is the time, I had an urgent call from Drew that their caregiver had just called my house looking for me. My mom was having a seizure and the caregiver was very concerned. My mom was in the bathroom when it happened. She passed out and fell into the bathtub. My dad immediately went home to help.

The caregiver told me (not Drew thankfully!) that she really thought my mom might be dying, but then my mom came to again. The caregiver was very scared. My mom is prone to seizures and takes anti-seizure medication. However, this was the first seizure that the caregiver had witnessed. My mom is okay now, just resting. I don't know that the caregiver will want to witness another episode like this as she is not trained medically for this type of situation. I would not want to witness a seizure either! Today's episode may help move my dad in the direction of the Alzheimer's unit.

Dad is supposed to be calling the elder law attorney to start the Medicaid proceedings and discuss his financial matters. The nursing home will need to come to their house and do an evaluation of my mom to see if she is still able to be placed in the Alzheimer's Unit. They did say the best way to have her placed is if she comes directly from a three day hospital stay.

My sister, Michelle, was going to call and talk with my dad tonight to encourage him that it is okay to check out the nursing home. She works with a lady who used to work in that field and really recommended the unit we visited today. That person told Michelle that if Mom could get in now, we needed to do it while we still can. The facility we looked at has a really good program. I hope my dad will have peace about pursuing this. It seems right.

I did have to have a discussion with Drew and Luke today about all this. Luke asked if people die from dementia, so I thought this is the best time to have that conversation with them. They had known about the nursing home visit with my dad today and that it was important.

Drew had an interesting perspective on it all. He said he wondered if the whole reason he was sick and had to come home from school was so he could be here to get the call to help Grandma. I thought that was a really mature perspective for a 14 year old boy! While I hated he had to take that call, I'm glad he saw it as a blessing!

March 4, 2010

Mom will be having an evaluation for the Alzheimer's Unit on Saturday. This is done at their house. This will determine if she would fit in their Alzheimer's unit or need to be placed in the general nursing population. I don't think Dad would be open to that. Dad talks with his lawyer on Friday morning about the Medicaid filing and will begin that process. He's talking with his pastor today. A lot hinges on this evaluation on Saturday.

I learned yesterday that the unit does have a bed available right now which is highly unusual. Usually there is a waiting list of a few people. I told Dad that maybe God is allowing all these things to come to a head this week- visit, bed open, mom's seizure, caregiver's stress, one of the worst days ever (Mom ripped down their shower curtain and pulled the shampoo holder off the wall in the shower yesterday!) - to move us in this direction. Maybe, we should begin walking down this path until God closes the doors. If God is making a way, we don't want to miss it. I trust that, if this is not best, He will close the doors.

We are not saying anything to Grandma until after Saturday. If Mom does get approved, I would think we would have to move pretty quickly on the available bed. I would guess that Mom would need to go to the hospital probably on Monday. We haven't talked with her doctor. Dad wanted to wait until after the evaluation.

I just don't know right now what the next week holds!

March 6, 2010

Today was the evaluation today for the Alzheimer's Unit. We will find out the answer tomorrow. My mom did have a good day, but we are really uncertain and not real hopeful that she will get in. The director seemed concerned with the amount of supervision and assistance my mom needs just walking at this point. The recent falls and seizure have really affected how she gets around. We would still prefer that she gets into this unit. My dad has resigned himself that this is best for my mom at this time. If approved, she would go to the hospital Monday or Tuesday and be placed in the unit at the end of the week.

My dad is not open to the regular nursing home care. He can't seem to process that she needs that yet, even though she does. We did discuss other options if she is not accepted. However, I would still prefer that she goes to the nursing home. I told him we could use it as therapy to see if they could help her with her walking, using walker/wheelchair, eating, etc. Yet, ultimately he must make the decision.

His relationship with the caregiver has improved since earlier in the week when they both were at their wits' end. They both need more time away from my mom. His plan does include that during the day, but evening and weekend care is still needed at home.

I had asked some friends to be praying for us about this transition. It has been amazing how I have seen God work this week. I'm hopeful that He is still working, no matter what happens.

Tonight the kids have an obligation for school. So I think Randy and I are going out to dinner to just take a break! Tomorrow, I will clean the house because Bill and Sammie (my in-laws) are coming from Texas on Monday night. It will be so nice to have them here so I can help out wherever I'm needed with my parents.

March 7, 2010

Well, we are waiting now until at least Tuesday. I spoke with the Alzheimer's Unit Director today. She said she still has to talk with the Director of Nursing who is off tomorrow. So, the wait for an answer continues!

March 9, 2010

My dad heard back today from the Alzheimer's Unit. They are concerned about the impulsiveness attached with my mom's type of dementia. They have asked for her to come for four hours and be observed in their unit. My dad will drop her off Wednesday from 10:30am-2:30pm. They will get to see how she reacts, eats, walks around, etc. Still praying this will work out!

March 10, 2010

My mom was accepted into the Alzheimer's Unit! YEAH!!!! At this point, Mom will be admitted to the hospital on Monday. Someone will need to be with her around the clock. On Thursday she will be moved to the nursing home.

I saw her right after her visit to the nursing home today. She said the food was good. She liked playing Bingo. She thought the people were nice and that the facility was clean.

She overheard us talking about her going to the hospital and asked why. We told her that she would be evaluated for help in walking and doing things she needs and she said ok. Hopefully her positive attitude will continue!

My dad said he is okay and thinks this is best. However, he is sad. During some time alone with him, my dad just began to cry. He curled up on his bed in a fetal position and just cried like a baby. He said, "It would have been easier if she had died than to put her in a nursing home. I NEVER wanted to do this. She never wanted this!"

I've never seen him like this. It was so sad to watch! He was always so strong. At times, I feel like I am killing him while I'm encouraging him to make these decisions for Mom. I know, in the end, this is best. He needs a break. Yet, it is so difficult to watch.

My grandma (her mom) was told today. She was obviously upset, but she knew that at some point we would need to do this. She is glad Mom will get the care she needs. Yet, no mother should have to face this with her child!

So many have shown us love by praying and caring for us. I know my dad and my family really appreciates and feels their prayers. We are thankful to God for this answer to prayer!

March 17, 2010

My mom was admitted to the hospital on Monday. The doctor had us go through the emergency room to be admitted. Although the hospital was really full and it took most of the day to get a bed, we made it! My mom was really quite calm in the ER and in her room on Monday. Tuesday, we noticed she had not even been out of bed and seemed more confused, so we did have her sit in the chair for most of the afternoon and went for two walks in the hall. That seemed to help her disposition a bit!

The hospital is requiring 24-hour supervision while she is there. So we are all taking turns. The good news is the hospital is providing a sitter for the midnight shift! I'm going in today and tomorrow at 7am to cover the mornings.

Yesterday (Tuesday), my dad and I went to the nursing home to complete the paperwork and begin setting up her room. My dad is going to take a dresser over this morning and finish setting it up. He seems resigned to the fact this is best for Mom, but it is really hard on him.

Before going to the nursing home, we went out for breakfast. I mentioned something about telling the boys that we need to remember who Mom was and hold on to those memories. Dad broke down and started crying in the restaurant. I felt so bad! My dad would never do that before; I know he is just emotionally raw right now.

The nursing home did tell us that for the first few weeks we will need to limit our visits until she is adjusted. They want her to acclimate to her new environment. I'm guessing that will be difficult for my dad too.

We've been asking people to pray that Mom remains calm and at peace (oh, and us too!) What a transition this is for us all!

March 18, 2010

Today, my mom was discharged from the hospital and admitted to the nursing home.

Dad seemed to be doing better today. He said he was at peace about it and resolved that this was best for Mom. Mom was REALLY sleepy today. When we left the nursing home about

1:30pm, she was going to lay down for a nap. I'm hoping that after actually resting she will be more alert.

Dad had to run medications for tonight to the nursing home. Her medicine is ordered but didn't arrive yet. They think they will get her medications by morning.

The room looks nice. She has 2 roommates: Mary and Gladys. Mary is very friendly, in her 70's, spry and very mobile. Gladys is not doing well, seems like she is in her 80's, and entering hospice, so Mom will probably be getting a new roommate soon.

Mom does need to improve or she could get transferred to a different area. They did change a few medications at the hospital so it might be that or it could just be a bad night of sleep or lots of motion. I'm hoping tomorrow is better.

She will be getting physical therapy and occupational therapy at the nursing home. The doctor requested it. Dad did have to select a new doctor for the nursing home; so, he used the one that his doctor recommended from the list.

They had all the patients outside in their courtyard today enjoying the sunshine. What a beautiful day!

Today is Grandma Niccum's birthday. Mom and Dad called her on Tuesday and sang Happy Birthday. Grandma said she was so surprised Mom knew all the words. Grandma loved that!

March 19, 2010

After we had left my mom yesterday, I mentioned to my dad that people were praying for Mom to have peace during the transition. He laughed and said, "You got to be careful what you pray for!" My mom was so peaceful; she totally slept the time away! We could not keep her alert. When we were ready to leave the hospital, my dad told her to wake up and open her eyes. She said, "No, I like to sleep this way!" LOL!!!

That being said, we did get her transferred over to the nursing home. She would answer questions (with her eyes shut!). She did wake up to eat lunch. After lunch, they helped her into her bed for a nap. We heard she was alert and talking with some of the ladies while reading the newspaper later in the afternoon. She did not seem to be reacting badly to being in a new environment. She was told she would be going to a new place that would offer her therapy to try to walk better and make her life easier. She seemed okay with that.

My dad seemed to do well yesterday too. He did not really want to leave the nursing home. After some time had passed, I suggested it might be good for Mom to actually take a nap and that would be a good time for us to go. He seemed okay with that. He did have to go back to drop off some medications last night; but he didn't go in and talk with my mom.

We did go to lunch after leaving the nursing home. Dad said he was resigned to the fact that this was best for Mom. He did pray at lunch that "people would not forget about Ruthie as she is at the nursing home." I think going to the hospital might have been worse than the nursing home, as the hospital really signaled Mom is not coming back home.

They did say that usually they ask the family not to come for a few weeks. However, with how my mom was reacting, they thought Dad could try to come and see her. If she wants to leave or has a bad reaction when he is there, he would then have to stay away for a while. He plans on going over this afternoon for an hour or so to see my mom.

We have made plans to go to my sister's house in Ft. Wayne next week on Thursday and Friday. All the sisters and grandkids will be together. I am sure it will be hard for my dad to fully enjoy himself when he thinks about Mom not being there, but I hope he will have a great time just being Grandpa!

We have felt the prayers of others. In fact, we have really been at peace as we have seen God move on our behalf. We're hopeful and prayerful that Mom will adjust well to being in the nursing home. We hope that the physical and occupational therapies can help with her daily struggles. She seemed to regress so much at the hospital.

4 THE ALZHEIMER'S UNIT

March 19, 2010

I spoke with Dad today. He was looking for more nightgowns to take to Mom. Not only did he find the gowns, he found his missing money clip with $171. in it! It had been missing for over six months. I'm sure he will be finding a lot of things as he begins to go through Mom's things!

He was told that she was doing well this morning and that she had a good night last night. He is planning to go see her. I hope she reacts well so that he can visit her and not have to stay away for a few weeks. I think that would be awfully hard on him.

March 21, 2010

Today was my first day to visit the nursing home. I feel like the wind has been knocked out of my sails!

I arrived to a lady in a wheelchair yelling at the man in the wheelchair in front of her. I had no idea what she needed or wanted, just that she was not happy! I blew it off.

I walked to the back of the nursing home and then entered the Alzheimer's Unit. My mom was in the main dining room supposedly watching TV, but really sleeping in her chair. She said hello but then went back to talking nonsense and picking at things.

I met Toni, a lovely lady who had strokes and now has no short term memory. She told me about buying her house in town for $9,000 in the 1950's. Then she told me the story all over again! She was very nice. The whole time my mom picked at Toni's sweater and her arm.

I asked a nurses aide to help Mom into her bed for a nap, since she was already sleeping in her chair. I learned that on Mom's first night, the aide had a really rough night with my mom. My mom kept getting up and down. Not a good thing since she is a fall risk. Ugh.... I hope she makes it in this area.

Her roommate, Gladys, is dying from Alzheimer's. Her family is at the nursing home often. The other day, hospice workers were there too. That is how I know she is at the end. Today I saw her feet - they were purple and black. She is on oxygen and does not get out of her bed. I don't want to see my mom go like that. It's so sad.

Today, I also talked with my dad. Yesterday, he was so encouraged by Mom. She had even been walking again with assistance. Today, she is not walking at all. I guess right after my dad left today, Mom fell. They called to let him know. Oh, I feel for him! He said that, on Friday, he really wondered if he had done the right thing.

Today, I wondered if I had done the right thing in recommending the nursing home! Mom has deteriorated so much in the last few weeks. Some say she might rally and improve once she gets adjusted. This is just very hard. I know it was the right decision. God made it very clear, opening door after door. Now, it is just hard to walk this out. They say it is harder on the family than on the person with dementia. At least the patient forgets. It is always before our eyes.

March 23, 2010

My second visit to the nursing home was better. No weird people in the hall. Mom was more herself. She even commented that she was starting to feel more like herself. I guess she realized she was not right!

I got there a few minutes before lunch. They were all in the main dining hall answering trivia questions. My mom did get the question "what is a dermatologist?" correct ~ skin doctor. She knows her doctors!

I was able to help Mom with her lunch until my dad got there. Their former caregiver came with him today. It was good to see her. It seems like so long since I saw her at the hospital last Tuesday. So much has transpired since then.

I feel so much better after seeing my mom today. She was awake and alert. She was not as tired and lethargic. Although she was still confused, she was not as confused and out of touch as she had been recently. I'm not ready for that to be permanent yet!

April 3, 2010

This last week has been an emotional roller coaster! Last Saturday, March 27th, was my 40th birthday. I thought it would be good for me to go see my mom at the nursing home. I was hoping that Mom might remember something about me being born when I was there. Also, I've been hoping she would fit in at the nursing home.

When I arrived, the residents were all in the dining areas waiting for lunch. My mom was sitting at the table and talking, but she was far from there mentally. Her eyes were closed, and she was hallucinating. I said to the other ladies at the table, "she is just not herself." One lady said, "She's always like this!" With the tone, I just knew my mom doesn't even fit in here! She is so different than the others. They can feed themselves, stay awake, and most can hold a conversation. They just don't remember things!

I mentioned that it was my birthday, but Mom didn't respond at all. I miss my mom!

I left really discouraged again, wondering if we did the right thing in placing her there. The staff is great, but she has regressed so much!

On Sunday, I shared with my Sunday school class that I don't feel I was prepared for the emotional side of this transition. It has been so draining. I am finding the time involved in going to see her, communicating with my sisters, and caring for my dad is just mushrooming! I cannot seem to calm down and breathe at all.

On Sunday afternoon, I went on an overnight prayer retreat with a friend. During that time, my friend asked me to write down all that I am currently doing on slips of paper. She had me put down the amount of time I spend each week on each category. I was amazed to calculate I am spending an additional ten hours or more each week caring for my mom. I was involved in so many areas and something had to give! I met with my pastor and asked to be removed of many of my responsibilities at church during this time. I want no regrets when we get to the other side of this dementia. Although I can serve others later, I can only serve my mother now.

My dad began investigating about her medicine. She was so much worse than at home. We did find out the nurse was giving her three Ativan pills a day. The doctor had said three, as needed, but she was only taking one pill per day at home. We wonder if reducing the quantity of the Ativan pills will help with her alertness. Ativan is a powerful drug used for her anxiety issues.

Michelle went to the nursing home for the first time on Monday. She had a really hard time. Mom was so confused and did not even know her. Mom kept calling Michelle "That Girl". That is not real welcoming when you are the daughter. This was the first time Mom didn't know Michelle. It is just an awful feeling to not be remembered by your mother!

Tuesday, Grandma Niccum called. She wants to come up and see Mom because "if something happened, I couldn't live with myself if I didn't see her at least one more time." That is hard to hear! We decided that it was best for Grandma to come on Thursday and stay a few days. We were just praying for a miracle that Mom would improve!

Wednesday afternoon I had a little extra time. So I went by the nursing home. I got there during sing-a-long hour. The aide needed to tend to another resident. I told the aide I could lead a few songs. They were using a hymnal, so I knew many of the songs.

After the first song, a gentleman said "That was beautiful. Sing another." He continued to say that after each song that he liked! One lady in the Alzheimer's Unit attended the same church as my family when I was a child. She does not recognize me now. When she knew the song, she would look at me and say, "I love you." At the end, she said, "I love you. What's your name? I really love you." That was so sweet!

Thursday morning came. It was the first day without the morning Ativan. Mom was so much better! When Grandma arrived, Dad asked Mom who was there and she said, "My Mother." Oh, my grandma's heart warmed. Grandma had been so scared of what she would see. She said she was surprised at how distressed my mom looked but she was so glad Mom recognized her and Uncle Howard. Funny thing was Mom didn't know who her husband was that day!

On Friday, Mom did even better! I think there is something to removing the extra Ativan. She is doing so much better! She is so much more alert and awake. The difference is just amazing!

Mom got her hair done for the first time at the nursing home. She looked so nice. Must have made her feel better. She used to get it done every week. I think Dad is going to start doing this more often.

Grandma was even happier with how much Mom did on Friday. Grandma had brought a wrapped box of chocolate covered cherries. This was a favorite gift she would often give to my mom. She held out the gift and without opening it Mom said it was "sweet cherries". Yes, she still knows her chocolate! This made Grandma feel so good!

Today is the day before Easter. We decided to have our dinner on Saturday instead of Sunday this year. Easter Sunday is so busy with special church services, breakfasts and the like. Both Grandma Foster and Grandma Niccum were able to be here today, making our time extra special! In addition, Dad was able to pick up Mom for her first trip out.

None of us knew how she would do. Yet, she seemed to do very well! She enjoyed her dinner, and she loved the roski cookies. She kept eating "One more for the road!" So glad we could have this time with her.

A funny thing was she kept talking about how she was going to have a baby. She told us about her contractions and how soon it would be time. You just never know what is going on with her or how her brain is working. I decided to loosen the safety belt on her wheelchair and the contractions seemed to go away! ☺

My dad asked Michelle and me to take Mom back to the nursing home while he took Grandma Niccum to meet Uncle Howard. I was quite apprehensive about how Mom would react going back. Would she fight us on this or go willingly? The only problem we had was getting her into the wheelchair from the car. She didn't trust the chair behind her and thought she was going to fall.

We got her back to her room and into her nicer wheelchair. She seemed content. We walked her into the dining room where she visited with the ladies at her dinner table. Michelle and I gave her a kiss and left. She did not react at all.

April 10, 2010

Well, this week has been interesting. Dad received a call on Monday that the director of the Alzheimer's Unit wanted to meet with us the next day. Would they kick Mom out of the unit? They had 30 days to do that. Oh, no!

Dad and I arrived for the meeting and were surprised by all the participants. Mom's physical therapists, her nursing supervisor, a dietician and the director were all there. It was a little intimidating!

The therapists both commented how much better Mom is doing, especially since the medication change. They said they think she is really funny. I don't remember her having a great sense of humor, but she must now!

The dietician talked about trying to get my mom feeding herself at least 75% of the meal each day. They are going to introduce some more finger foods so she can better feed herself.

The nurse commented how concerned she was at the number of medications Mom takes. Dad needs to get an appointment at the University of Chicago to have all this reviewed. She has two depression medications, plus two or three memory drugs- so much duplication. If she needs them all, that is great! But it does seem like the medications could be doing more harm than good.

The director spoke to us also. Mom needs to be able to remove her safety belt on command and eat without assistance in order to stay in the unit. There was the "heavy" of it. If she isn't able to do these things, she will be moved out of the Alzheimer's Unit into the general nursing home population. I hope she can learn to take the belt off and on - but only at the appropriate times. I would hate to see her fall again.

I do not know if there will ever be a normal routine again. It seems like as soon as we adjust to one thing, there is something else that must be done! YIKES!

On Friday, I visited again. When I arrived, there was a lady singing and playing the banjo in the general dining room. I took Mom down to hear her. She seemed to enjoy it. I learned they have "Happy Hour" every Friday afternoon. They have a live musician and snacks. I think we might try to come to this program more often.

May 13, 2010

Well, we are now at week eight of the nursing home Alzheimer's Unit. A few days ago, the physical therapist stopped me and told me that Mom is not progressing in therapy any longer. She is being dropped from therapy. Today was her last day.

A real significance in all this is, that without progression or improvement, Medicare stops paying. It will soon be private pay if there is no change in her medical condition. She is not responding to the therapy by showing improvement.

It is just sad how this disease keeps taking and taking. Seems like soon there will be nothing left. I know that is not true, but reality is so stark these days.

Tomorrow, Dad and I are taking Mom to her neurologist at the University Of Chicago Hospitals. We are hoping that they can adjust her medications or at least let us know if the changes we are seeing are strictly the disease progressing. The Alzheimer's Unit director told my dad that my mom has the most mind altering medications of any of their residents EVER. That is scary!

Last weekend was Mother's Day. I was asked to write a brief article for our church's women's newsletter. Here it is:

Honoring my mother this Mother's Day will be totally different than any other year! In the past, we would visit my parent's home, share a meal, and give her flowers. This year, we will drive to a nursing home, walk to the far corner, and enter a locked Alzheimer's unit. Six weeks ago, our family had to make the most loving and difficult choice: to provide the special care Mom needed. We now celebrate her feeding herself, remembering who we are, and her just being with us. Life is precious!

Even though she may not always know her daughters, I still know my mother. I choose to honor the great and caring woman she was, celebrate the victories she has now, and have hope of her glorious future in heaven. I love you, Mom (Ruth Ann Foster).

Mother's Day was different. Angie's family came, as well as Michelle and Rebekah, Randy, Drew and Luke. We decided to do dinner at the nursing home instead of trying to go out to eat. Mom has so much difficulty getting in and out of the car.

It was nice to all be together. We missed Jerry who was working. Yet, it was very surreal. This was the first time Angie had been to the nursing home or seen Mom in this very compromised state. Mom was so tired and lethargic during her party. She couldn't feed herself or even open her presents. But she was there! I guess that is a blessing.

Last week on Monday, May 10th, I started a Breakfast Club for daughters who have a parent with dementia-related illness. There were four of us. One lady's mom is in the dying stage so we listened and each shared as we could. I think this will be good to get together with other daughters and be able to share openly since we are all on the same journey. I keep saying this is the group no one wants to join, but they come out of need. I hope everything we are learning is not wasted.

JULIE HAYDEN

5 THE B-WING

June 1, 2010

Well, this is the entry I've been avoiding for 10 days. On Friday, May 21st, Mom was moved out of the Alzheimer's Unit and into a "skilled care and behavioral issues unit." B-wing is so different from the Alzheimer's Unit. *[horrible name]*

First there is the noise! The "yellers" are on this wing. There is constant calling out by the residents. Just so sad!

Then, there's the smell. Since almost all of the residents are incontinent, the poopy diaper smell fills the air. I don't think there would be any way to not have some smell with that many adult diapers. It greets you as you walk past the laundry and garbage bins in the hallways.

The staff: They are different than on the other unit. I hear that they do not stay working on this unit as long, and I think I understand why. They do not seem to be as interactive with the residents either. They don't have the time to spend one on one like the other unit staff was able to do. There are so many resident needs they have to address. I heard there is less staff per resident in this area. Seems like there should be more, not less. They don't seem to interact as much with each resident individually, leaving them just to sit in their chairs and stare off into space. The residents are all lined up in front of the nurse's station.

I will say that her room is nicer and larger. She has just one roommate, who is really quiet and sleeps a lot. Her roommate does have the window view. Mom has plenty of room for her dresser and chair in this room. It is funny how all of Mom's possessions have been pared down to one dresser and chair!

It is hard to go to the nursing home again. I just HATE this unit!!!! I know Mom needs more care, but I dislike seeing that displayed with every resident. They all are very needy!

I hate this disease and what it is doing to my mother, my father and even me!

July 29, 2010

Sometimes, I hate writing in this diary. Putting it all down in ink makes it all very real and I cannot deny what is going on.

My dad and I did go look at another nursing home. But for now, he wants to keep Mom where she is. Some things have improved: they are working on the smell, the staff seems to be more interactive with us, and my mom really likes some of the aides. The staff does seem to really care about Mom and us. So I guess that is all good. No place is perfect.

We learned the reason the patients sit in their wheelchairs by the nurse's station is so that the nurses and aides can care for them the best. It allows the staff to interact more with the residents as they

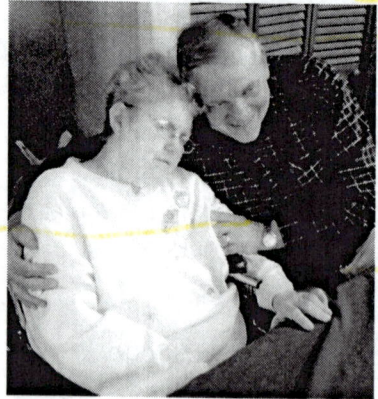

pass by. Funny how our perceptions can be so wrong initially! I thought that was a bad thing; not a good thing.

There is a table by the nurse's station with baby toys, games, and magazines on it. Different residents will sit there to read or play. It is strange how grown people are unable to do a simple toddler maze or matching game. It is also odd to watch grown women dressing and rocking baby dolls. This is all just is not right.

On June 25th, my mom celebrated her 63rd birthday. The Saturday before, Michelle and Angie and their families came for a visit. We took Mom and Dad out for lunch to a local restaurant. Mom seemed to really enjoy herself and laughed a lot. At one point, Mom called Angie by her name which made Angie's day! It was good to see Mom have such a nice time.

As her birthday approached, Dad and I decided to take her to lunch for her actual birthday. That Friday morning, I decided she needed a party, so I began calling some of their friends. Funny thing - my dad was calling their friends (THE SAME ONES) at the exact same time. Neither of us had talked about it. She had a grand party at her favorite Chinese restaurant! She really seemed to enjoy it!

Since then, there has not been a lot of change in her. She is more alert right now, but still not making any cognitive improvements.

However, I think I am imploding. I have held it together for so long that I seem to be busting at the seams. Can't seem to stop it either!

While on vacation a few weeks ago with Randy's family, my volcano of emotions erupted on my father-in-law. Right now, when things are out of my control, I get very agitated and short. I am just not a nice person. I do not like how I react. I just can't handle anything beyond my control. Randy's dad was concerned about me and lovingly was asking if everything was okay. It was more than I could handle; I was face to face with my anger and concern about my mom's condition.

I quickly excused myself from the conversation and just started bawling. I didn't know if I could stop! It went on for almost an hour, off and on. Then yesterday, it happened again; although, not so severe.

Mom usually is happy. Yesterday, I was curling her hair and putting make up on her when all of a sudden she just started crying. I tried to ask her what was wrong. All Mom could get out was "I can't..." I have no idea what she was upset about. She kept saying something about her mom and dad. I hate this disease!!!! As I left the nursing home, I was crying too.

I'm starting to let more people know about my issues with this, but it is not easy being vulnerable. I think most people don't understand; and some just don't want to know. I did confide in two friends last night. I know they will pray, and I guess that is what I need most right now.

December 6, 2010

I just have not been able to write. There has been so much change in Mom and in my life that I haven't wanted to write.

In October, Grandma Foster (my dad's mother) had a stroke. For three weeks, Grandma struggled - up one day, down the next. Finally, she passed peacefully to glory! She is with the Lord. No more struggle!

At the funeral dinner, my cousin commented just how fast everything had happened. Michelle and I commented what a blessing it was that it was quick. Having watched Mom's struggle for the past five years, three weeks seemed like a huge blessing! I guess without the path we have walked with dementia, I would never have seen it this way either.

Mom joined us for Thanksgiving at my house. I was amazed how well she did. She seemed to enjoy the day. Dad didn't want it to end. I can't imagine what that must be like.

One neat story: towards the end of our time together, I had the thought that maybe she could play the piano. So I wheeled her up to it, and she played the piano! She was playing melodies with her right hand. She struggled a bit putting two hands together, but I was amazed how well she did! Hmmm....maybe it is still there somewhere.

I started a job! I'm the interim worship leader at Family Bible Church, filling in while their worship pastor is on a sabbatical. The thought that came to me is that in the midst of death, God is giving me something life giving. I'm really enjoying the work. What a blessing from God!

Yet, I'm struggling with making the time to visit Mom. There always seems to be one more thing I can or need to do. I don't know why I seem to be avoiding going to see Mom these days. It makes me mad at myself!

Christmas is fast approaching. We are hoping to have Mom come to our family Christmas on the 18th. Hopefully she will do as well as on Thanksgiving. Her mom and family should be here too!

On December 19th I'm planning a program at the nursing home for Family Bible Church. Hope it is enjoyable to the people there!

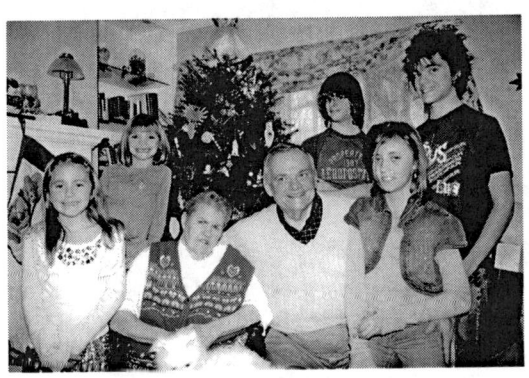

January 1, 2011

Well, Christmas has come and gone. With it came challenges with Mom. What do you take her to? What do we not have her attend? How do we process the guilt we feel celebrating without her? What do you even give her for a Christmas gift?

She did come to our family Christmas on December 18th at my house. Unfortunately, it was not a great day for her. She was confused and not with it. She seemed very distant.

We had planned to get Mom to my house before anyone else arrived. That way, we'd have time to fix her hair, change her clothes and get her settled. But, it didn't work that way.

Before Mom arrived, her sister, Connie, and her mom, Grandma Niccum, arrived at my house. We had to work to get Mom into my house with her wheelchair. It was hard to watch her sister. This was the first time she had seen Mom in a year. I could tell my aunt's mind was flooding with thoughts- so much to process all at once!

Mom did seem to laugh and enjoy all the great food! I gave her a piece of her favorite - Sugar Cream Pie. Oddly, she did not like it at all! She thought it tasted terrible. Go figure! Everything is different!

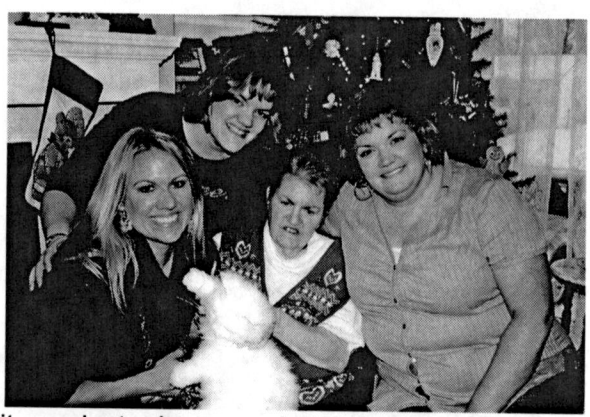

Dad found a Fur Real cat for her. It looks like the cat we had when I was growing up. Mom held the toy cat and petted it and combed its hair. She didn't want to let it go. She was very protective of it. While I loved seeing her enjoy her gift so much, it was just a huge reminder that the Mom I knew would understand that this is only a toy. Today, however, my mom does not. To her, this is her new cat. She loves to pet it and has it on her lap while she sits in her wheelchair. I'm glad she has the company!

The next evening, I was able to lead a group from Family Bible Church to go caroling and perform a Christmas program at the nursing home. It seemed to go well. Mom and Dad went with us as we caroled to the Alzheimer's Unit. It was great to see the people

Mom first met at the nursing home. They were so welcoming to our group!

We did not have Mom join us at my sister's house on Christmas day. There were too many stairs, and Michelle's house is too far away. While we all knew it was not possible to have Mom join us on Christmas, it seemed very odd. So much is so different now.

Yesterday, I went with Dad to the nursing home. When we arrived, one of our family friends greeted us and mentioned that their mother was being transferred from the Alzheimer's Unit to the B Wing. This is such a hard transition for the patient and the families! She had been in the Alzheimer's Unit for over 10 years. When I saw the mother, she was just so confused and crying. It made us so sad! I hate this disease!

I am really enjoying my new job. It is so wonderful to feel so alive again! It is hard to believe it has only been a month. I love what I do: creating a worship set and then worshipping the King of Kings with a group of amazing people! God is good to me, giving me life in the midst of death and hope in the midst of sorrow!

Tomorrow morning, we are singing *I Will Rise*, a song talking about the hope of resurrection from the dead. This world is not it! Death is not final! We have eternity with Christ! What a joy to remember this in the midst of dementia! My mom has a hope beyond this disease! She has an eternity with Christ! No pain, no sickness, no more death, no more tears! Hallelujah!!!

JULIE HAYDEN

6 THE END HAS COME

September 23, 2011

Silence is not always golden. Nine months have gone by since my last entry. While I've often thought of writing, I just could not do it. The slow steady decline has increased to a rapid race to the finish and I have not wanted to acknowledge the inevitable.

In March, my birthday came and went again. Even my dad did not remember. Birthdays were always my mom's thing! She had loved buying the perfect gifts and sending the perfect card! While I wasn't upset at my dad, I was upset at dementia and the realization that my mom had no idea who I was or of her daughter's special day. When I told my dad, he was so apologetic about missing it. I know it was not intentional. He just always relied on my mom for those things.

My mom's disease has started to waste her body away. When she entered the nursing home she weighed about 185 pounds. Initially, she had lost a few pounds, but her weight had stabilized around 160. In the late spring, we started to notice that all her clothes were getting too large for her. In June, we took her to the doctor and realized she was down to 136 pounds! No wonder her extra large and extra, extra large clothes did not fit any more!

This week, my dad and I went to a local church's garage sale and purchased a whole new wardrobe for her in her new size – small and medium. We got it all for just $27! It is odd to think that she did not pick out one item in her closet anymore! She always loved picking out new clothes. I think she would like what we got her, but she can't tell us that.

That visit in June to her neurologist was the first inkling of what is now coming. Her doctor is so good - so professional and yet caring. Throughout the appointment, she just looked at my mother with sad eyes. The doctor's look was so different than on our previous visits. And then she said, "You never know what might happen. Do you have all of your paperwork in order?" I knew then that the doctor was seeing what we feared. We were moving more into the end stage of the dementia, and it would become more apparent very soon!

Over the spring and summer, Mom had a series of urinary tract infections. During this time, she became more withdrawn and more agitated. She would dehydrate and need fluids. Once she ended up in the hospital for a few days while they gave her fluids and IV antibiotics.

When I went to visit at the hospital, I was shocked by what I saw. She looked so small and frail in the bed. I told Randy, my husband, that I didn't know what would happen next. So, I was shocked and

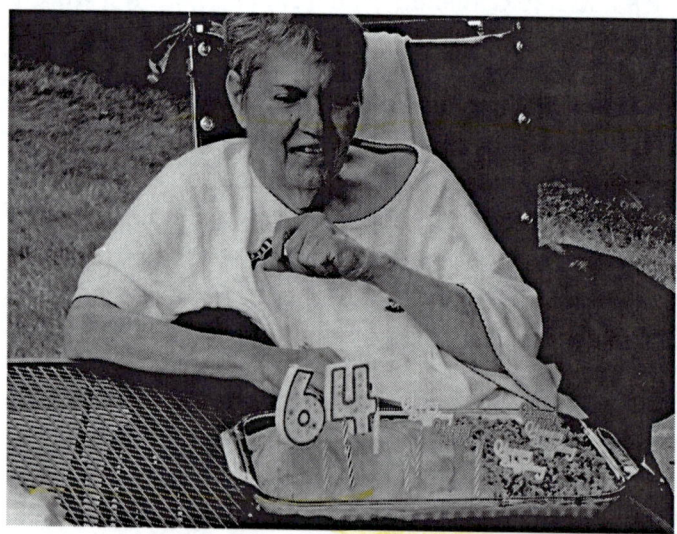

amazed when she was sent back to the nursing home the next day.

Her 64th birthday was in June. I had wanted to not to be in town that day. Friends of ours had a son getting married that day and I wanted to escape by attending his wedding. As the date got closer, I knew I needed to stay and celebrate Mom's birthday; no matter how hard it would be.

We had a party for her outside the nursing home. Grandma Niccum and Uncle Howard came. It was a beautiful day outside! Mom had a pretty good day too. We brought in pizza and cake. We took lots of pictures and celebrated this milestone!

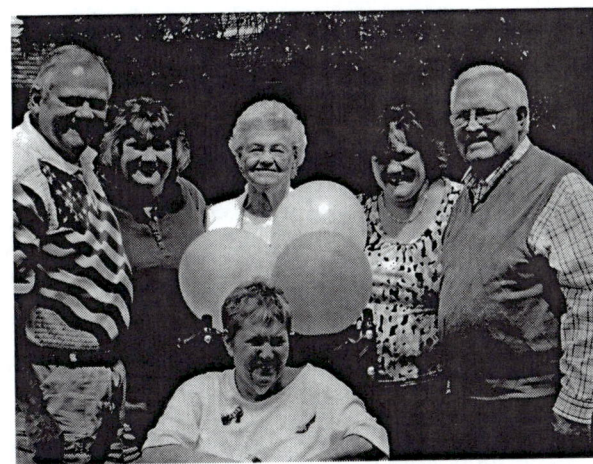

During her latest infection in August, one of the nurses at the nursing home approached my dad. She mentioned to him that it might be time to consider hospice care. My dad was devastated. Did she only have days to live? Was this the very end? What does this mean?

I had been out of town for three days. When I returned home, two of my parent's friends told me how upset my dad was about my mom's condition. All I knew was that she had an infection. Suddenly, we had to consider hospice care for Mom!

My dad and I began talking about the possibility of hospice. What would be the pros and cons of this decision? The main question that kept coming up was: while we did not want any extreme measures, what do we think is extreme? What about a feeding tube? Hydration? We already had a do not resuscitate order. Is it moral to not do a feeding tube? Do we want her to starve to death?

After about two weeks talking with just my dad and me, we planned a family meeting. Michelle and Angie's families were coming over for a visit so we made time to talk about these issues together. We had some mixed emotions. We wrestled with what we were all comfortable with. We even called the Alzheimer's 24 Hour Helpline for information as we made our decisions and weighed our options. Where did we want Mom to spend her last days: at home, in a nursing home or a hospice center? We ultimately decided to pursue the hospice service.

In September, we visited Mom's neurologist again in Chicago. This time we brought up to the doctor our decision to pursue hospice care for Mom. She mentioned she thought that would be wonderful for Mom. Mom had lost an additional 13 pounds in 3 months – now weighing only 123 pounds. Mom just seems to be withering away!

Dad and I met with the two hospice services that come to the nursing home. While many of the services were the same (2-3 nursing visits each week, 2-3 additional bath aides, social worker for the family and chaplain services), how they administer pain medications varied and only one offers the possibility of a family center where we can stay with her in a private room during her final days. We did choose the one that gave us the most options to keep her comfortable and the family together. It has been a very clinical approach this week to the hospice entrance. We've weighed and discussed. We have contemplated and frustrated! We have thought and prayed.

I called the hospice center to arrange for us to begin the process the following week. We were previously led to believe that we had a few months -nothing urgent. I had gone to lunch with some friends and the hospice in-take nurse called me back wanting to admit her that afternoon. I told them how the family wanted to wait till the next weekend when we could all be in town. The nurse told me, "We think it is best to admit her today." There was the strong implication that waiting a week might be beyond what we have. What were they seeing that we are not seeing? This was the first we'd heard about death being imminent.

Today, my dad had to make the very difficult phone call to Grandma Niccum, her mother. While it was not a huge shock to Grandma, no mother is ever ready to hear that their daughter is entering hospice. Dad said they had a good cry together over the phone. She has decided to come up on Monday. She wants to make sure to see her daughter again. These visits are hard and so sad! I can not imagine what Grandma must be feeling!

This week, we also had a scare. For two days, she really didn't want to eat or drink. The staff believes she may have had a seizure. They called my dad to say she was unresponsive. While her vital signs were okay, she would not respond or wake up. It made us realize that this really could be anytime.

I don't want to miss an opportunity just because it is so painfully hard. In the past, I had hoped that the end would come for Mom with a quick seizure or that she would quietly die in her sleep. I did not want to walk this road. I did not want to get to this point of making these decisions and watching her body waste away.

Part of me wishes I could cry more, but most of me does not want to let myself. If I start, I don't know I can stop!

October 20, 2011

Hard to believe all that has transpired in just one month's time! My mom is now a resident of heaven. On Thursday, October 6, around 3:15 am, Mom slipped peacefully into eternity.

Right after we signed her up for hospice, things began to decline quickly! The eating was the most notable. She began to not swallow. Mom had always eaten well – solid foods, not ground food. For a few days, she would not swallow anything - no medicine, no water, no food, and no chocolate!

Then, we had a great weekend. Michelle and her daughter, Rebekah, came. Angie and her girls, Madi and Macy, came to visit too. Grandma Niccum came up to stay until the end. Angie was able to get Mom to eat two whole meals – one on Saturday and one on Sunday. No one else could get her to eat, but Angie did!

We began taking turns saying our goodbyes. Each of us would sneak a few private moments with Mom just to tell her how much we loved her and that it was okay for her to go ahead to Heaven. We did not want her to suffer any more. Yet, facing the reality of the end being near was hard! Many tears were shed by all of us, and even Mom had some tears as well.

That Saturday evening, the family gathered at my house to talk about funeral homes and plan the funeral. What an awkward time! We were trying to figure out if there was a message we would like to present through Mom's service. Did we want the funeral in the morning or evening? What songs should be sung?

The sisters decided to pre-record the song, *Blessings* by Laura Story, to be played at the funeral. We had a good time practicing and singing together. We couldn't remember a time as adults that we all sang together. My dad just loved the song recording! We played it for Mom on Monday and for any one else who came to visit her. When Mom heard it for the first time, she attentively listened to the song and kind of smiled.

On Monday, one of her life-long friends came for a visit. Her friend came early and got there before my dad or me. She quickly found Mom's room and checked it, but didn't see Ruth Ann. She went and asked the nurse where Ruth Ann was. The nurse said she had just put her in her room. Her friend argued that there was someone in there, but it wasn't Ruth Ann. Unfortunately it was! My mom's best friend did not even recognize her. Mom had lost so much weight. Her eyes were glassy and glazing over. Her mouth was open most of the time in an awkward way. She was back to not eating or drinking anything.

Her friend felt awful at not even recognizing Mom. They had been so close for so many years! She was shocked at the changes since her last visit. She lives about an hour away; so she doesn't get here often.

Grandma had decided to stay here for a while, waiting to see if Mom would get better or if this was the end. What a hard thing to watch - your daughter slipping away! I can not even imagine.

Michelle, Gina (my sister's best friend) and Grandma stayed with Mom on Tuesday while Dad and I went to the funeral home to make arrangements. We were still being told one or two weeks at this point. We needed to determine which funeral home we would be using before she passed or we could have to pay additional fees to transfer the body later. (All things you don't want to think about!) I had contacted all the funeral homes in town to collect the information and presented the information to Dad. We thought we had settled on one, but Dad needed to make the final decision. Since Mom was in good hands, we went and picked out a casket, made pre-arrangements and determined who would handle her services.

That is such an odd thing! And an expensive one too! No one wants to use their services, but you have too. Which vault? Which casket? Burial or cremation? Open or closed casket? Private or public services? And then the flowers.... The list just goes on and on.

The chaplain for the hospice service came on Tuesday afternoon. I am glad we made it back in time for his visit. He played guitar and sang some old hymns. We all sang along. Even Mom was trying to sing along as she mouthed the beginning words to *The Old Rugged Cross*. We also sang *How Great Thou Art* and *In the Garden*. What a nice time we all had together singing! Grandma's great alto parts added so much. Some tears were shed that day.

Grandma and Dad had been coming back each night to try to feed Mom. We had determined with the hospice nurse that if she was not able to swallow the thickened water, we should not be trying the food. She was storing food in the back of her mouth – not a pleasant thing. She could not swallow anything – not even her very important anti-seizure medicine or Parkinson's pills. This had us all very concerned!

Tuesday night, Dad and Grandma were not able to get her to eat at all. They also noticed her breathing seemed different. It was a little shallower.

Tuesday night, my in-laws arrived from Texas. They were coming for their fall visit. We had been planning this trip for months! They were going to help Randy replace some doors and windows, as well as drywall a room in our house, getting ready for a new kitchen and dining room next spring. It is always good when they come. We all enjoy their company.

On Wednesday morning, I got up and finished a few things around the house that needed to be done. Randy had the day off to help his dad at the house. I left around 9:30am for just another day at the nursing home.

As I was pulling into the nursing home parking lot, I had this sinking feeling in the pit of my stomach. I knew that this day would be the last time I would visit my mom at the nursing home. I didn't have anything to base it on other than God sometimes would speak to my heart to prepare me for what was to come.

When I walked into the nursing home, my mom wasn't sitting by the nurses' station. She had been spending more time in her room. So I went to her room. When I saw her, I thought, "Is she still alive? Is she even breathing?" I was really upset. Her breathing was really quiet and then she would have short bursts of rapid breathing, like she was hyperventilating.

I went and talked with her nurse. She said she was thinking one or two days at most! What a shock! The nurse mentioned she had seen a huge change over the last day.

My dad was supposed to be there any minute. As I sat at my mom's bedside, I was just all choked up. This was it! It could be anytime! I watched out the window waiting for any sign of my grandma and Dad. I was so scared that he would not get there and that I would be alone with her when she passed.

I saw them enter, but they did not come to the room right away. I could hear my dad's booming voice, but he was not in our wing. I went out in the hall to search for him. I was scared. When he saw my face, he knew it wasn't good.

As soon as he and Grandma saw Mom they both broke down crying. We all knew it was bad! The nursing home was calling the hospice nurse to see if Mom could be transferred to the hospice center right away. They have private rooms there and better options of ways to make Mom comfortable.

The hospice nurse arrived about an hour later. A new social worker was with her too. They both were very nice. She evaluated my mom and said she did not see signs of active dying. She would talk with the hospice center to see if we could get approval to move Mom; but she warned us it could be up to two more weeks like this and if Mom did not progress towards death, she would be returned to the nursing home.

We weighed our options and, in the end, decided to go with the nursing home's evaluation to move her. The nursing home staff had told us they felt this was the end, and if we could move her, to do it! If the patient is too near death, they are unable move them. We did not want to miss our opportunity.

Dad, the social worker and I quickly started putting her stuff together. Things to take to the hospice center. Stuff to go to his house. The nursing home policy was that we needed to remove her belongings within 24 hours of leaving the facility. Randy and my father-in-law were called to come get the stuff and take it to my dad's house while the rest of us went to the hospice center.

Grandma and I got some lunch from the nursing home staff. They were so kind to bring us a lunch tray with bean soup and a sandwich. I did not know when we would get to eat again. And I knew if I did not eat something then, we would have more problems on our hands later.

In between all the packing, eating, crying, and decision-making, we made phone calls to Michelle and Angie. Both made plans to drop everything and come over. The nursing home was still saying 1-2 days max while the hospice workers were saying 1-2 weeks.

When the transport ambulance arrived, the driver mentioned someone from the family could ride along. So Grandma decided to go with them. Then they said, "Just so you know, if something happens, we do not stop until we get to the hospice center." UGGHHH! That cut like a knife!

Mom left with Grandma and the ambulance drivers. Then Dad took off. I waited a few minutes until Michelle, Randy and my father-in-law all arrived. We loaded up Mom's stuff, said goodbye to the nurses who had become like family to us, and began the trek to the hospice center.

It was a surreal drive. Knowing you are going to watch someone die! How do you prepare yourself for that? I made a few phone calls just asking for prayer. I shed a few tears too.

When I got to the hospice center, Mom was in her room and the staff was getting her evaluated. We were asked to wait in the waiting room. I learned that, on the way to the center, the back ambulance worker began asking how much longer they had. I guess Mom did not have a good ride there.

When we were able to go in to see Mom, it hit us all again. She was in the bed; the room was lovely and very peaceful. There was a reclining loveseat, some other chairs, the hospital bed, TV, and a bathroom. Mom looked so weak and frail. She now had oxygen to help her breathe.

With each new person that entered, the look of "the end is near" was apparent. Angie got there about 3:30pm. She immediately broke into tears. It was so apparent to us the changes in Mom's breathing and appearance in just the last few days; even over the last few hours. Michelle leaned over to Mom and said, "All your babies are here now." Michelle said she saw a tear run down Mom's cheek.

For the last week or so, we couldn't hear or understand what Mom was trying to say. Initially, she would try to talk, but it was so faint we could not make it out. It was so hard to know that the last things she would try to say to us we could not be heard.

It had seemed that Mom knew what was happening too. So often over the last six months, she had seemed so out of it. Yet, in the last few weeks, it seemed she understood that she was near the end. She reacted when each of us said our goodbyes. She was agitated during the hospice in-take meetings and even yelled at one point. I have to believe she knew what was happening, at least on some level.

That day in the hospice center we shared stories and laughed. Many people came to visit: Bill and Sammie Hayden (my in-laws), Aunt Suzi, Drew, Luke, and Randy. My parent's pastor came. The hospice social worker came back to check on us. Gina came and stayed with us – even running out to get dinner for us.

Drew and Luke came to say their goodbyes that evening. It was hard and awkward for them as 15 year olds, but they did it. Grandpa helped them through it, explaining along the way what was happening with Grandma and how our faith in God gives us hope. The boys were so amazed that Grandpa was so concerned about them during their final time with Grandma. It really made an impression on them.

Right after they left, Mom had a series of three small convulsions. That really scared me! I was sitting next to her bed, and I jumped! The nurse was able to give Mom something that would help her be calmer. She did not have any more seizures or convulsions.

All afternoon, we had been told that it could be weeks and that we did not need to stay the night. Angie began making plans to go back to her home the next day. She needed to wrap up some things and prepare for an extended stay the next week. So, she volunteered to spend the night with Mom. We did not want her to be alone. Yet, Angie said she was fine and, if anything happened, she would be okay since she is a nurse.

I could not believe we were going home Wednesday night. I kept asking my dad and Grandma, "Are you sure you want to go home?" My dad kept saying that the hospice nurse said it would be at least a week, maybe two. We needed our rest.

So around 10:00 pm, we began our goodnights, not knowing they would be our goodbyes. I remember telling Mom that I loved her and that I would see her soon. We all walked out together and left. Only Angie stayed.

I came home. I put together an emergency bag of clothes, books, and personal items. I set out a clean change of clothes in case I got a call and needed to leave quickly. Then I sent this email to my friends:

Hello!

My mom was moved to the Hospice center today. The nursing home nurses felt the end was in the next 24-48 hours. Hospice felt it might be longer. She is now on oxygen and being given medicine to keep her comfortable. We are really glad to be at the center. It is very nice. Her breathing has become quite shallow with some rapid breathing patches. She also has had some convulsions, which are disturbing to us. I'll keep you posted as I'm able. My sister Angie is spending the night tonight. She is a nurse and thought we should all get some sleep tonight. She came in this afternoon.

All the sisters were there tonight along with my grandma (her mom). Randy, Drew and Luke came for a while with Randy's parents who are visiting from out of state. My parent's pastor was there for a while too. A few others came by too. We had a lot of great story telling. My dad is always the story teller.

Thanks for your prayers! We are feeling them. This morning was very difficult. My dad, grandma and I all knew just looking at her that things had changed drastically overnight. Once she was at the hospice center, we were able to relax a bit more as they were able to get her medicines quickly in her system (she has not been able to swallow anything so she wasn't receiving any medicine since Sunday)

Thanks for your prayers!

Pat was my mom's nurse all afternoon. She was very compassionate to my mom and all of us! She got off work around 9:00 pm and then finished her charts. As she was in the parking lot getting ready to leave at 11:00 pm, she felt she needed to come back inside and tell my sister that they were wrong. It was not going to be weeks, just days.

Angie texted me that and said she was getting ready for bed. I was still awake, struggling to fall asleep. I just couldn't believe I was at home and not there, but knew it was ok.

At around 3:15 am, the phone rang. Angie was crying and saying, "Her breathing has changed. If you want to see her again, come now!" I hung up and jumped into action, quickly putting on the clothes I had laid out the night before. My dad called to make sure I knew to come.

As I drove there, I thought, "Will she even be alive when I get there?" The answer I seemed to know was that she would not, but that seemed so far from what we had been told.

I remember debating in the car whether to take in the bag I had made with books and stuff for a day of waiting. I decided I should bring it in, just in case I needed it and didn't get a chance to leave. However, I really didn't think I would need it.

I entered my code and walked through the secured doors. It was 3:45 am. I opened the door to my mom's room and saw Angie sitting at the head of the bed stroking my mom's hair. She said,

"She's gone." Tears were streaming down Angie's cheeks. I was the first to arrive.

Angie said that she had fallen asleep around midnight. At 2:00 am the night nurse came and checked Mom and there were no major changes. Angie was awakened at about 3:10 am because she did not hear breathing. She reached over and felt Mom's heart beating. She called the nurse, and then quickly called Dad, myself and Michelle. Before the nurse could run and grab her stethoscope, it was done. Mom had passed from this life to eternal life. Angie had called Dad back so he knew that Mom was gone and not to rush to get there. Then, she took a minute and prayed. She called Michelle back and told her as well.

It was very surreal when I got there. Mom's oxygen was still on and I could hear it blowing. It was so confusing to me in my tired, emotional state. Angie removed it, and we sat in the room with Mom's body waiting for Dad and Grandma to arrive. Michelle was not able to come back during the night as there was no one to care for her daughter, Rebekah, since her husband was out of town.

When Dad and Grandma arrived, the tears flowed again. Angie and the nurse had wrapped Mom in warm blankets so her body wouldn't be cold when Dad got there. They both went up and kissed and hugged her ~ crying all the while.

Dad had us all gather around her. We held hands above her body and each prayed a prayer, thanking God for her life and releasing her to His presence. It was a very moving time!

We were told we could stay with her as long as we liked. We stayed in the room with her about an hour. Then, we checked with the nurse about contacting the funeral home. The nurse said there were some preparations they needed to make. So we left the room and went to the waiting room for a while.

While in the lounge, Dad told stories about when each of us girls was born. We laughed a little remembering while drinking a cup of strong coffee.

When we came back to the room, Mom was now in a paper gown. We began to pull together the things we had brought there just a day before thinking we'd be there for two weeks. After about a half hour, the funeral directors arrived to take Mom's body.

They gave us a few minutes with her. We each said our goodbyes again. I have never been able to touch a dead person. I had wondered how it would be with Mom. I still could not do it. I felt guilty about it, but I could not touch her. In my mind, she was gone. She was in heaven.

It is funny how we all react differently to death. I had been secretly praying that I would not have to be there when Mom passed. I knew that most likely I would be there, and I would have if Dad had asked us to stay. But, I just really did not want to be. We did not know what that would look like, and we really feared Mom might have a seizure that would cause her death. I guess God answered my secret prayer.

After our goodbyes, we gathered all of Mom's stuff and quietly walked out of the building. What a weird walk! Three cars. Four people. Bags of stuff. Loads of heartbreak. We decided to go home, shower, and meet for breakfast. So much had happened already - and it was only 6:00 am.

I knew I would be home before the kids left for school. As I drove home, I began to try to figure out how to tell them. I started to cry on the drive home. I had been feeling strong and happy for Mom up until that point. It was beginning to hit me.

I came in the house and just told the kids what happened. In many ways, there was no outward reaction. We had all been expecting it, and yet, it all seemed unreal too. I decided to take a shower and drive the kids to school. It gave them a few more minutes that morning to process and deal with their day.

I sent a quick email before we headed out that morning:

What a sight my mother is beholding today! At 3:15 I got a call to come back quickly. My sister, Angie, who is a nurse, stayed the night last night. Before any of us could get there, Mom quietly and peacefully drew her last breath here and entered Heaven. My sister was sleeping but awoke right before noticing the change. Before the nurse could even check, Mom completed her journey.

We are praising God for her life and yet mourning at the same time. We are so grateful for so much of the family being with her yesterday and enjoying the day, as well as a very peaceful exit from this life....

Thanks for your prayers over the years for my mom and your prayers for my family now.

Love you all!

After dropping the boys at school, I drove to Dad's house. We were all meeting there and then going to breakfast.

The phone lines were popping at Dad's that morning. Everyone making phone calls, letting people know that Mom had passed. People in multiple rooms on home phones and cell phones, all talking at the same time. I began to go through the photo books to begin selecting pictures for the video for the funeral.

The weekend before, we had sat down as a family and discussed what we wanted for the funeral. We had a few songs in mind. One song was called *Walking Her Home,* and we wanted a video of pictures in the background. The song spoke of a husband walking through life and death hand in hand with his wife.

Later, we went to breakfast. All the time we were at the restaurant, my phone kept ringing. It was Randy, then my dad's pastor, and more calls kept coming. Michelle joined us for breakfast. It was nice to have her there.

Michelle shared about telling her daughter, Rebekah. She told her she had some good news to share about Grandma. She told

Rebekah that Jesus came and got Grandma last night. Grandma is all better now. Rebekah was so excited; she wanted to know how she could know that when she died she would go to Heaven with Jesus too. Then, Rebekah broke out into a song they sing at their church: "Grandma found the happy side of life.....with Jesus by her side, Grandma found the happy side of life!" Out of the mouth of babes! What a wonderful perspective!

After our breakfast, we all trekked over to the florist. I was grateful to see my friend, Nancy. She was so kind to us! We all had so little sleep and were just running on adrenaline by 11:00 am when we got there. We quickly decided on a casket spray in autumn colors. It was so good to see a friend and share for the first time what had happened.

Then, we went back to the house for round two of picture-searching and waiting for the next appointment. We were just about to leave for the funeral home when we realized we needed Mom's clothes and jewelry. We quickly found the funeral dress, but all of Mom's good jewelry was GONE! Dad put it away for safe keeping, and now we could not find it anywhere.

We got to the appointment late – and without the jewelry! By 1:00 pm, we were all slap happy! I don't think the mortician knew what he was in for. We laughed over my dad's constant edits to the obituary text. After about five revisions, it was right and we were on our way.

We went back to the house again to look for jewelry and go through pictures. My Mom's last caregiver stopped by the house for a few minutes. Then, a longtime family friend came by with a delicious dinner. It was so nice to see her and have her join us for a meal.

By the time I got home, I was beat!!! Luckily another friend had brought a meal for my family too. I came home and visited with our company. Then, I went to bed. Yet, I could not sleep. I just kept thinking about all that needed to be done before Sunday's visitation and funeral.

Saturday, we were celebrating Macy's birthday with a party in Ft. Wayne. It was good to go and celebrate family. Yet, it was so weird to think that we were having a party one day and a funeral the next!

On Sunday, I decided to go to church. I figured I might as well since we didn't have to be at the church for the funeral until 1:00 pm. I was so caught off guard when the first person came up and gave me a hug. I hadn't realized how that would feel. I was so choked up and teary-eyed. It was a hard morning.

The visitation and funeral were both being held at my parent's church on Sunday. I could not believe the flowers and all the people! There was a line out the sanctuary for most of the time - so many people came!

I was so surprised by all the friends who came to support me who had never met my parents. What a blessing! People came from all the places were I served: prayer group friends, Daughters of Dementia Breakfast Club ladies, church friends from Liberty Bible, Family Bible, and Portage Christian Fellowship. So many friends showing us love and caring! My heart was warmed.

The service was great – for a funeral. It really seemed more like a celebration of her life. It all came off just like we planned. The boys and I did *The Family Song* (see Appendix A). The granddaughters sang *Amazing Grace*. The slides and songs were perfect! All three of Mom's daughters, Dad, Rebekah, Luke and one of my mom's friends all spoke at the funeral. The pastor gave a great message of encouragement.

My mom was a special lady. We had said we wanted the funeral to be a celebration of her life, and God went above and beyond our wildest imaginations. As we were walking the casket to the hearse, we noticed that someone in town was lighting off fireworks – the big kind used in 4th of July celebrations – at exactly that moment! The fireworks would explode right over top the church steeple. What an interesting way of celebrating a life well lived!

On Monday morning, the burial service was held at the cemetery for close friends and family. The family arrived a little early and while we were talking about the flowers and plants, my Meniere's disease acted up. I was SO dizzy! My sisters noticed the sudden change in my walking. I immediately took my medication!

(Care giving can have a very negative effect on the health of the caregiver. In many cases, the primary caregiver dies before the person they are caring for!!!! For me, my health decline was seen when I was diagnosed with Meniere's disease during Mom's time at the nursing home. While it is under control now, without a miracle, I will carry this reminder with me the rest of my life.)

At the cemetery, Uncle Howard sang the hymn, *What a Day that Will Be*. My parent's former pastor shared stories about them. Prayers were offered. We moved to the burial site and encircled the final resting place and prayed again.

Leaving the cemetery felt so odd. It was a "what do we do now" moment. It seemed so weird to be leaving her there. We had planned a luncheon that day for close friends and family at a local restaurant, so at least we had a somewhere to go.

As we were leaving the restaurant, Dad called his three girls together. He told us how proud he was of us, how much he loved us, and how we truly honored our mom. It was a special moment for all of us.

By the time I got home at 2:30 pm, I was wiped out! I really wanted some time to myself. I felt so conflicted since we had company, and I had not spent any time with them. I didn't know what end was up.

Randy mentioned that, since I had been care-giving for the last six years, Mom's death was kind of like suddenly being unemployed and your Mom dying both at the same time. I had made caring for my family my first priority. Some ministry and job opportunities had been put on hold while we waited for the end to come. And now that it had, where do I go from here?

That's the question I keep asking now. What should I be doing? Should I be working? Should I just take some time? What is my next step? And how do I even begin again? Some opportunities are gone. Some will never come around again. Everything seems so unclear and unknown.

7 GOING FORWARD

November 22, 2011

Thanksgiving is in two days. This will be the first holiday without the hope of Mom attending. It still feels very surreal.

I've been talking about going to their house and getting Mom's china for the dinner. She had the most beautiful china pattern. Silver edges with pink flowers. It was a gift to her from her grandmother for her hope chest when she was sixteen.

I keep thinking I need to go get it. Yet, I can not motivate to do it. It seems so final. She really will not be here with us this year. Last year, she was here – and it was difficult, but at least she was here!

She always liked the jellied cranberry sauce. The rest of us like the whole berry type. It seemed odd not to purchase the jellied sauce this year. I thought about it the whole time I was in the store. It is funny the things that bring you pause.

Over the weekend, my sons were involved in a play at their school. This year's production was *Flowers for Algernon*. The kids did a phenomenal job. The play is about a middle age man, Charly Gordon, who was mentally handicapped from birth. He has an operation that makes him super intelligent. He learns afterwards that he can not maintain his new mental skills and you see (and feel) his demise to his former self.

As I watched Charly's battle to keep his mental faculties, I thought of how the dementia affected my mom. I remembered her fear and frustration as she began to realize that she could not remember things and how she was unable to do what she once was able to do. I wondered how scary that must have been for her, knowing that she frequently could not even put into words how she felt or what she feared.

Dementia stinks!

November 30, 2011

Thanksgiving is over, and I am glad! My dad brought me the special china. He said it was not a problem. That was until he tried to get it out. It ended up being tough for him too.

We had a good actual Thanksgiving Day. My grandma was able to come up for the weekend. We had a nice visit. This is the first Thanksgiving she has spent with us in decades. It was so nice to have her here.

On Saturday, I had a blue day. I was on the verge of tears all day. I went to our local home improvement store. In the parking lot, I talked with a friend who is losing her job on January 1st. As we stood outside in the wind, we both had tears streaming down our face as we discussed our losses. It is strange where and when grief hits you!

I still do not know where we are to go from here! How do you begin again? I am starting to think about some ministry activities again. For the first time since Mom passed, I am going to lead worship for an area meeting on Saturday. I am looking forward to serving in this way again!

Life must go on! Life is for living!

8 LESSONS LEARNED

These six years have been a huge learning time for me. I learned a lot about myself, my family, dementia, living, and dying. I do believe that God allows us to go through things so that we are drawn closer to Him and also so we may help others who are facing similar situations. Instead of just rescuing us from our lives, He chooses to join us in the journey.

Here are some of the things I've learned along the way.

We Need Each Other

The path of dementia is hard and filled with potholes! You need others! As you saw from my diary, I frequently turned to a small group of friends for prayer and support. I was honest with them about where I was and where my mom was in her disease. They would pray for me when I could not. There were times when I just had no strength – but they did!

I would encourage you to find a small group of friends that you can be really honest and vulnerable with about your struggles with dementia. Find those that will pray, speak truth to you when you need it, and care for you.

This could be a church group – a Sunday school class, a small group, or prayer group. It could be close friends. It may be family members not immediately affected by caring for the person with dementia. My in-laws were a great support to me throughout this process.

Join a support group or create one of your own. Some of the best encouragement and insight came from others who had walked this road ahead of me. I have built relationships that I will have for the rest of my life.

Resources Are Available in Your Community

Take advantage of the resources in your community. There are many resources available, but sometimes connecting with them can be a challenge.

Start with the Alzheimer's Association. (www.alz.org or 800-272-3900) From their website, you can get connected with state or area coordinators that know the resources available in your area. Many local areas offer free resource guides which list available services in your area.

The Alzheimer's Association also offers many free seminars and informational meetings. They have the latest information available and love to share it with others! They also coordinate support groups for the family members of people with Alzheimer's disease and other forms of dementia.

Other places to contact are your doctors, your area agency on aging representatives, senior centers, and your church. Frequently, there are resources available. You just have to find them!

Long-Term Care Workers Are Amazing!

As my mother's disease progressed, we began to realize just how amazing the nursing home staff was. They cared for her 24 hours a day. They were there when we could not be there. They spent more time daily with her than we were able to. They showed genuine concern and love towards her. One staff member even asked us if we would consider moving my mom to the hallway where she worked. She wanted to care for her!

It takes a special person to want to work in long-term health care. They are very giving individuals and deserve respect for what they do! Often, they are understaffed and overworked. Yet, they do their best to care for those in their charge. They not only care for the patients; they walk with the families as well.

If you have issues with the care your loved one is receiving, talk to those in charge. See if there can be changes made to meet your needs. We learned that as we praised them when praise was due, we were heard when change was needed as well.

If you have questions about your parent, talk to the nurses, talk to the aides, or meet with the social workers. They are all there to help you and walk with you through the disease process. They are a wealth of information! They desire to meet your family's needs.

Treat them the way you would want to be treated. Be nice to them. They might have patients yelling at them all day. Find ways to encourage and bless them.

Communication is a Key

Early in our disease process, we began having family meetings. This was a time when my dad and his daughters would sit and discuss what was going on with Mom. It gave us a chance to talk openly about changes in Mom's care, long-term planning, as well as care for my dad's needs. We could talk openly and come to agreement together about what was best for Mom. At each major milestone in her progression, we would schedule a family meeting.

At times these meetings would include others. Initially my mom was included in the discussions about her care. As time progressed we would have these meetings without her. Also, her mother, who is still alive, was included in the discussions as much as possible. Spouses were included in some discussions, but not in all. Their opinions were important but were given through the birth child.

With all of the stress and confusion dementia brings, the best thing you can do is to keep clear communication between all involved parties. So much can be clouded by the chaos of the disease. Protect the family relationships as much as possible. You will need them!

If you are unable to physically meet, get creative with your communication. Use a group email. Set a time and have a conference call. Have a facebook group for those who need to know. Find ways to keep open communication whenever possible.

Prepare for the Future

As soon as you are able, begin to prepare for the future. Set your financial house in order. Meet with an elder law attorney to prepare advanced directives for you and your loved one. Advanced directives are necessary for all adults – you never know when you might need this important paperwork!

Try to stay one step ahead of the disease in your preparations. While your loved one is still able to be on their own, begin to research what options are in your area for adult day care or in-home services. Know what your options are before it is an emotion-driven decision.

Discuss, as a family, your end-of-life decisions ahead of time. If your loved one is capable, get their input early on. Find out their wishes. What life saving measures do they want used? Is hospice an option? Where do they prefer to die?

As the disease progresses, decide on a funeral home and cemetery. Pre-plan the funeral with a funeral director. When you need this information later, it will already be completed.

My Path Is Not Your Path

While you may read my story and some aspects of it may parallel to your own, our journeys will be different. Every family's path is different. Every person progresses at different intervals and has different medical needs. What worked for our family may or may not work for you. This was my story, my path.

Listen to others and seek counsel, but make your own decisions.

At one point before placing my mom in a nursing facility, a friend shared about a bad experience with a nursing home. She felt that was the worst thing they did in caring for her mother. She felt it hastened her mother's death. At the time, we were just beginning to consider nursing home care. I took her words to heart, but weighed them against the other mitigating factors in our situation. We made our own decision.

Even within my family, my experience with Mom's dementia is different than either of my sisters' experiences. My dad's story would be different from mine. We each process things differently. We are all at different places in life and have different responsibilities.

Over the years of my mother's disease, I struggled with the responsibility I felt in caring for my mom and supporting my dad, while still balancing the needs of my own husband, children, home, and ministry. One of my sisters worked full-time, while the other sister lived out of the area. Their lives and family responsibilities were not the same as mine. They took different roles in the care of my mom.

You are only responsible for your own actions – not anyone else's actions. Only you can make decisions for yourself. Each person makes their own decision of what is best for their family. Support one another and do what you are able.

I was very grateful to have the full support of my husband. He was wonderful throughout the process. His role was to support me as I supported my parents. He would help behind the scenes, but he left visiting the nursing home and providing supervision to me. He was a great listener for me. He always encouraged me to do what I felt I needed to do. Yet, in love and wisdom, he would let me know when I needed to pull back and rest.

My children also were very supportive. They were nine years old when the dementia began. Over the years, they saw more of the disease than I ever wanted them to see. Many times, they would have to wait on something they needed or wanted while I tended to their grandmother. While they didn't always like it, they understood the importance of caring for family.

After my mom was in the nursing home, I would try to plan most of my visits without them. However, they would usually go with me at least once a month. I would try to make the trip special. We would plan our trip around an activity at the nursing home like a music performance or special meal. Sometimes we would make our own special activity by picking up milkshakes on the way. I knew it was hard for them to be there; so, I tried to keep their visits short.

I did also appreciate the closeness I gained with my father through our journey. Often, I would try to visit the nursing home when I knew he would be there. I think it made the visits better for both of us! I got to know him so much better through all the time we spent caring for my mom.

No Regrets

"I want to look back with no regrets." This was a phrase my sisters and I said often. This meant different things to each member of my family, but it was a theme we all tried to live by.

This belief in "No Regrets" became very real to me the last Christmas we had together before my mom entered the nursing home. As I looked forward to that holiday, I thought of it as if it could be our last Christmas. I invited my parents over more frequently. We went out driving to look at Christmas lights together as a family. We had an extra special dinner together on Christmas Eve. Whatever was in my heart to do, I did! I am so glad I did!

Dementia is a progressive disease. You never know when the next progression is going to come. Yet, be assured it will come! If it is in your heart to show love in some way to your parent and it is within your means to do so, do it! Don't wait - it might be too late!

Once my mom entered the nursing home, we tried to have at least one visitor a day for my mom. We would normally have a family member try to be there over the lunch hour to help feed her one meal a day. I would try to go about twice a week to visit. My dad was averaging being there 5-6 days a week. There were days that I did not want to go to the nursing home at all. As time progressed, it became harder and harder to visit all the time. I hated seeing the deterioration of my mother. In those times, I would think, "If something happened today, would I wish I had gone? Would I wish I had baked those cookies she loved? Would I wish I had taken that time and put her needs above my own?"

It is always good to show love to those that we care for! This is good for all the relationships in our lives - not just those suffering from dementia.

It's Hard! Don't Feel Guilty!

Watching your loved one's health fail is hard! It is very painful! The parent you knew seems to be gone, and you don't recognize the person who is left in their body! There are days when you feel you cannot emotionally go there one more time – you cannot witness it without falling apart.

Please know your feelings are normal! It is normal to cry. It is normal to feel anger towards the disease. It is normal to need a break once in a while. It is normal to feel guilty for wanting that break.

Give yourself grace at times to release the emotions that are building within you. If you don't, you will implode. Schedule pressure releases in your life: coffee with a friend, a good movie where you can cry, a weekend away, a good night's sleep, etc. Keep spending time with God in His word and prayer.

Know that there will be times when you react poorly to your parent or others. When possible, apologize to them. Forgive yourself and receive God's forgiveness. Then, go on. No one is perfect. It is a hard transition to parent your parent!

It Is An "Is"

During the first year of my mom's dementia, she and I adopted a phrase: "It is what it is. This is just an 'is'!" What we could not change became an "is".

Barring a miracle, her dementia would not change. We could treat it; but it was not going away. We could not will it to be gone. Dementia, along with its byproducts, became an "is".

For example, early in her dementia, my mom wanted to drive. She hated that she was not being allowed to drive. Not being able to drive was an "is" for her. It was a fact that we could not change. She had to accept it and believe it to be true, all the while hoping that it might change in the future.

Because of the dementia, many things became an "is" for her: not driving, not being able to stay by herself, not remembering names, not wanting to be in crowds, not being able to cook, having to go to sitters and senior centers, etc.

For me, I had some issues that were an "is" too: my mom needed supervision, not being able to control my own schedule, receiving my mom's frequent calls in the middle of the night, watching her deteriorate, visiting her at the nursing home even when she did not know me or my name, thinking about her death, and putting aside some of my dreams to care for her. These were some of my issues to work through. I am sure everyone has their own issues to deal with.

What About God and Healing?

During her first hospitalization for dementia, I remember sitting up throughout the night. She had to have supervision around the clock. I had just started reading a book on divine healing. I thought this dementia was just a blip on the radar screen of life. God was going to heal her instantaneously, and, then, we would be moving on to bigger and better things. I thought that her healing would make an excellent testimony and who knows what God would do from there. HA!

Reading my story, you know God chose to heal her over five years later..... by taking her to Heaven. In the process, He taught me a whole lot about His healing and His grace to walk with us through tough situations. Sometimes the greatest miracle we are given is the grace needed every day to walk the path before us.

I still believe God can do anything. He could have chosen to heal my mother. Yet, He chose to draw close to us, change us, and give us grace for each day, each hour, each moment. I long for the day I hear testimony of God's supernatural healing in the life of someone with Alzheimer's or dementia. I still pray for healing for others. I know He can do it. Yet, for now, I rest in His goodness and His grace today. God is sovereign. Some things will remain an "is".

It would be easy to doubt that God is good when you think about dementia. However, day after day, we saw how He provided and cared for all of us including my mother. This was not the plan we had for her; yet, we could trust that He was still with us. He promises to never leave us or forsake us. We saw that to be true! Even when my mom couldn't remember Him, He remembered her! What a good God we have!

You Are Not Alone

I hope that through this retelling of my story with my mom, you will know that you are not alone. You may be on what seems a lonely path, but you are not alone. There are many others who are walking similar paths all around you.

Even more, there is One who wants to walk with you. His name is Jesus! The Bible tells us that though He was God, He became a man just like us. He knew heartache for those He loved. He wept with His friends and He desires to be near you! He loves you!

Let's pray together:

Dear Lord,

Thank You for my friend who is reading this book. Thank You that You are near to the broken hearted; that You comfort those who mourn; that You give strength to the weary.

I thank You, Jesus, for providing an answer for our sin that separates us from God. Thank you for dying in my place and paying my penalty for sin. I receive you as my Lord and Savior today.

I pray that Your Holy Spirit would fill each of us this today with Your peace and Your presence. May we all have the comfort of knowing that You never leave us nor forsake us. In our weakness, we see You are strong.

Thank You for the wisdom You give to your children when we call on Your name. Give us Your grace to handle every situation we may face with our loved ones. Wrap us in Your loving arms.

In Jesus name-

Amen.

The LORD is near to the brokenhearted and saves the crushed in spirit.

~ Psalm 34:18

He gives power to the faint, and to him who has no might he increases strength. Even youths shall faint and be weary, and young men shall fall exhausted; but they who wait for the LORD shall renew their strength; they shall mount up with wings like eagles; they shall run and not be weary; they shall walk and not faint.

~ Isaiah 40:29-31

"Come to me, all who labor and are heavy laden, and I will give you rest. Take my yoke upon you, and learn from me, for I am gentle and lowly in heart, and you will find rest for your souls. For my yoke is easy, and my burden is light."

~ Matthew 11:28-30

JULIE HAYDEN

ADDITIONAL STORIES

APPENDIX A – BILL'S STORY
(MY DAD)

APPENDIX B- ANGIE'S STORY
(MY SISTER)

APPENDIX C- RANDY'S STORY
(MY HUSBAND)

APPENDIX D- DREW'S STORY
(MY SON)

APPENDIX E- THE FAMILY SONG

JULIE HAYDEN

APPENDIX A – BILL'S STORY

By Bill Foster

It has been 8 months now since the Lord took Ruth Ann to her final reward. As I reflect back on this journey I walked along with Ruthie, I know this was not the retirement we had planned for. I often think back to that day 44 years ago when my bride & I exchanged our wedding vows to that line…"in sickness and in health". I surely never imagined how this would play out over the last six years or so. Friends would ask, "How were you able to go through such a trial and still continue to smile?" It was only through the strength of my God plus my faith in Him along with knowing that the love of my life would have been there for me if our roles had been reversed.

I often thought that Ruthie's passing could not come too soon; but, whenever it would come, it would be too soon. No one wants to see their loved one suffer and to steadily decline. This journey was a gradual one and I continued to discover how just a little smile or a sparkle in Ruthie's eye or her just holding my hand would bring such joy to me. I tried to visit virtually every day but I also knew that there were wonderful family members, caregivers and nurses who loved and cared for my loved one in my absence.

This journey we took together was a slow gradual progression which seemingly never got better. It was like walking 2 steps backward with only a step, here and there, where we would see a glimmer of hope. Then there came the day when Ruth Ann had to take those final steps alone and to leave us behind. In the end, we had a celebration of her life service where we were able to recall all the wonderful things she did and the inspiration she was to our family & friends.

God has a wonderful way of allowing us to remember far more of the great memories while clouding over those unpleasant ones. An example of this is my final remembrance of Ruthie is not of her last days but of her enjoying a lovely lunch spent with her mom, uncle, daughter & I. How she just beamed and smiled in enjoyment of her soup and sandwich even though she could not speak.

I was so thankful for my girls who were there to aid & carry me through those difficult times and the decisions we had to make on Ruth Ann's behalf. The family meetings were so beneficial especially because everyone seemed to be on the same page with regards to our loved one's care. Ruthie's mom, Dewala, and Uncle Howard were also such stalwarts through this entire ordeal. I hope I never have to experience the loss of one of my children. To witness a mother's love first-hand was a real inspiration to me and our entire family.

My mourning process really began at the time that I had to put Ruth Ann into the nursing home nearly 18 months before her death. I believe that was the toughest decision of my life. I retired four months earlier to be able to care for her full time, along with our live in caregiver. I knew how much Ruth Ann despised nursing homes and I felt that our caregiver and I could do the job. My daughters, on the other hand, were seeing the toll that Ruthie's full time care was taking from my own health. Thus, the decision, however unpleasant, had to be made.

Shortly thereafter, I noticed I was suffering the effects of depression. I decided on my own that I needed to find something productive to do with my spare time so I began to mow lawns for friends and my church. It was just the medicine I needed to fill the voids in my life.

I must also share with you that there is still life after the loss of the love of your life. I have been able to do some traveling which I so enjoyed. I have also begun a relationship with a wonderful lady who has once again brought joy and meaningfulness into my life. I do not harbor guilt over "would of's, could of's & should of's" with regards to Ruth Ann's care and, thus, I am at peace as I closed that chapter in my life and as I look forward to what God has in store for me in the future.

APPENDIX B – ANGIE'S STORY

By Angie McCoy

Silence…a sound that most mothers of two young daughters hold dear. A sound that we almost never hear but revel in every chance we get. No crying, no whining, no "she hit me," or even any breathing.

Wait…no breathing. Oh my…no breathing!

When I lay down I could not sleep, because all I could focus on was her breathing! Now, the oxygen machine was still pumping out the gift of life, but my mom was no longer taking it in. "Oh no!" I thought, jumping from the chair that I had strategically placed touching the side of her bed, so I could feel if she had another seizure. I could not have fallen asleep during my duty as her night watchman.

As I ran out of the dark room and into the dimly lit hallway, I seemed to be emerging out of the twilight area between sleep and consciousness. I felt like I was in a bad horror movie running from a predator. Instead, I was running to find a nurse to determine if my fears were indeed a reality. Even though I knew it was best, I was just not ready to let her go. I never will be. I just got here today - I need more time. After seconds passed that felt like hours, I found the night shift nurse who brought in the stethoscope to confirm that my mother had indeed passed on to a better life than the one she was living here on earth.

My fear and concern were not for my mom, but for my father and her mother, who were sleeping soundly at home. In my mind, this was not how she was supposed to go. She was supposed to pass away like in the movies or in a good gospel song that leaves you with tears streaming down your cheeks, surrounded by all her loved ones "walking her home." Is it my fault that I slept through the subtle changes that transported her from her earthly home to her heavenly one? Was she waiting until no one was watching to let go? Only God knows. What I do know is that everything happens for a reason, and I am just so glad that I was blessed enough to be the one there by her side at that moment. Since living away at a distance, I could not be there for the day-to-day care and keeping of my mom.

Distance is a blessing and a curse when caring for an ailing parent. I did not have my mom's illness and progression in my face on a constant basis, giving me the pain of watching the process of her deteriorating like a bad scene in slow motion. On the other hand, the guilt of not being able to be there for the small stuff like painting her nails or looking through picture books to remind her of her loved ones was overwhelming at times. There were days when I was so glad that I could forget that my mom had dementia and Parkinson's disease.

Forgetting was a luxury that my dad and Julie did not get since they were primarily in charge of her daily care. From a distance, I saw the love and devotion that they provided to her and knew that she was in the best possible care. Even though my background was in nursing, I could not have done a better job. Julie showed the patience of Job. Even though she was pushed way beyond her limits, she remained a loving and steadfast caregiver to my mom.

In addition to my sister's devotion, the unwavering trust that my mom put in my dad to care for her needs was matched by the untiring devotion my dad showed my mom in return. I knew when I saw my dad doing my mom's hair and makeup that they had a very special relationship. My dad had grown into his new role in life. They really found strength in each other through adversity. That strength came from their mutual faith in God; knowing that this was His plan for their lives even though they may not understand why.

My mom's struggle has taught me the importance of a God-centered life to ensure an eternity free of the suffering that may occur here on earth. According to Romans 5:3-5, "We also rejoice in our suffering, because we know that suffering produces perseverance, perseverance, character and character, hope. And hope does not disappoint us, because God has poured out His love into our hearts by the Holy Spirit whom He has given us." I continue to hope that this is not a final goodbye, but a goodbye for now until we all see Mom again in Heaven, where she will greet us with a smile, a laugh and a huge hug.

I love you, Mom!

JULIE HAYDEN

APPENDIX C – RANDY'S STORY

By Randy Hayden

As a spouse, it can be a helpless feeling to not be able to take the hurt away or even know how to try. I watched my wife endure the long-term agony of a disease that took her mother a little bit at a time, and I could do nothing to prevent it. It took me a long time to know how to best serve the needs of Julie as she walked through this journey.

I loved Ruth Ann. Julie's story gives a fantastic glimpse into Ruthie's personality and how she felt about others, but unless you knew her, the story may just be words to you. It was special to have her as my mother-in-law. She always wanted to know more about what I was doing. I hear stories of disdain that people have toward their own mothers-in-law. I have never been able to understand that; I loved my mother-in-law.

Many questions went through my mind: What was my role to be in this? As just one of the three sons-in-law, what right do I have to inject myself in the family discussions about Ruthie's care? Does the family need one more opinion about medications, doctors, nursing homes, therapy, or even legal matters? I struggled to find my niche in the journey.

As the journey progressed, I began to understand things a bit more. My role was to support my wife, to ensure that she had a healthy balance between caring for her mother and being properly engaged in her own immediate family. I was Julie's support system. As flawed as I was at it, my primary responsibility was to Julie. As the head of my household, I was to focus on the protection of my family.

It was helpful for me to be able to settle into this role because I function better when I know my scope and the expectations others have on me. I am a "black and white" thinker who does not find compassion as my default position. A long-term disease like Ruthie's in some ways has to become a way of life. It is a marathon. As a family, we had to find ways to remove ourselves from survival mode and live in a balanced healthy way. Our kids went through many of their crucial years of development during Ruthie's illness so we had to embrace our own family life.

Now that Ruth Ann is in the presence of the Lord, we have had time to revisit the journey with the wisdom we wished we had during the journey. She had a life well lived and well celebrated. Her funeral was an amazing testament to her contribution into the lives of so many and her faithfulness to God. For me, I look back with some regret because, at times, I did not have a clear understanding of the emotions Julie was dealing with while on the journey. Now, I wish that I had been more in tune with what she was dealing with each day. I have learned now that it is about more than logistical solutions. I have learned that a timely hug can be more helpful than a fantastic, well-conceived solution. This is something that I had to come to grips with after the fact. I appreciate my understanding and forgiving wife.

My respect for my father-in-law has grown immensely. He tenderly cared for his wife for so many years and learned so much about compassion along the way. He is a poster child for the "…in sickness and in health, until death do us part…" aspect of marriage. Well done, Bill.

Moreover, I have learned that God's grace is sufficient for us. He gives us strength when we are weak. We are nothing without Him.

APPENDIX D – DREW'S STORY

By Drew Hayden

I'm Drew Hayden; I'm the oldest son of Julie (the author) and Randy Hayden. I am also the oldest grandchild of Ruth and Bill Foster. I am now 16 years old. Luke, my brother, and I were the most unprotected of the grandchildren from my grandmother's dementia, because we were the oldest grandchildren and the closest to the situation. My brother and I are also really the only ones of the grandchildren that knew the old Grandma. The others were too young or too far away to have really known her, which is sad for them.

I don't have many memories of the old Grandma, but I do have some. I remember when she would come over in the morning to watch us before school. She would always bring glazed chocolate donuts. Those donuts have very special significance to me. Isn't it strange the things that we find meaningful later in life?

Another memory that I have with my pre-dementia Grandma is making cookies. Well, perhaps the better term is baking cookies. We didn't actually mix the ingredients for the dough or buy a mix and add eggs; we got the Pillsbury sugar cookies that come in a "log". We would role the "log" in sprinkles, cut the "log" into slices, and then put the slices on a cookie sheet to bake. I had done that so many times with Grandma that I didn't know how to make cookies any other way. When my mom wanted to MAKE cookies we told her that she was doing it wrong and that you do it the way Grandma did.

There is one time during the middle of my Grandma's dementia I will never forget. Grandpa, Grandma, Luke, and I went up to their trailer in Michigan for a good time of fishing and the like. Things quickly turned ugly, not because of my Grandma's dementia, but because my Grandpa hurt himself. While trying to get out of the boat on to the street below he got caught and somehow he hurt his ankle. We returned to the trailer to just relax after the events in town and someone spilled something. It got on the floor and both my Grandpa and Grandma rushed to clean it up. My Grandpa got a paper towel, put it on the ground and started cleaning it up with his foot, which pains him because he had hurt his ankle earlier that day. My Grandma being caring says she'll do it, but my Grandpa had things under control. Things escaladed from there until my Grandma blurted out "D@#^ it, Bill." My old Grandma would never have dared cussing in front of my brother or me, but the disease had taken a hold and she was losing her filter. From that moment on, I knew things would never be the same. The Grandma I had known was no more.

My Grandpa's ankle continued to hurt and we thought that there was a possibility that he might have broken his leg, so we went to the hospital to get it check out. It turned out that he was fine and he hadn't broken his leg.

There was an entry in the book were I had come home from school sick and had received a call from the caregiver that Grandma had had a seizure and I needed to forward the message. As was said in the book, I did feel that God had me come home from school sick to get that call because there is no such thing as coincidences.

During the transition to the nursing home I was hoping that they would find a nursing home because of the tension that was growing in my Grandpa's life and my Mom's from having to watch Grandma 24/7. The nursing home was a hard decision but I agreed with it all the way and supported her placement in a nursing home. After my grandma was put in the nursing home, the health of my grandpa increased dramatically. He no longer looked tired or fatigued, and he had more energy. Grandpa visited Grandma almost every single day at the nursing home, which blew me away - the love that he had for her even though she didn't know who he was.

The Alzheimer's Ward was very nice, but the B wing was not so great. My Grandma went from the best part of the nursing home to the worst part of the nursing home. Every time I went to the nursing home I tried to smile because I didn't think that the people there saw smiling faces that often.

When she was transferred to hospice care, I was amazed at how nice it was. I also barely recognized my grandma. When saying my goodbyes, my grandpa talked about this analogy that the end of life is like a boat sailing of into the horizon, but how on the other side the boat is coming closer to shore. That struck a chord and I will probably remember that till I'm in that situation.

When I was told that my grandma had died I didn't really have a reaction physically or a huge one emotionally. To some readers that may seem strange and heartless, but the fact of the matter is that my grandma, as I had known her, had been gone for almost 2 years. I miss the Grandma I knew as a child. I will remember the fun times we had together.

APPENDIX E - THE FAMILY SONG

By Julie Hayden

My parents were from Christian homes that taught them right from wrong

My grandparents all served Jesus,

Grandma praised the Lord in song.

Mom gave her heart to Jesus and with Christ she always stayed

As a college man, Dad saw the way

And he bowed his head and prayed.

Well, they were married with three little girls

And they did the best they knew

With little money, but with lots of love

We always did make do

We never did without what we really needed most

For God was always with us and in Him we would boast.

So I'm grateful for the family God placed me in

Mom and Dad, they loved Jesus

And they kept us far from sin

My grandmas had a depth of faith throughout the thick and thin

Oh, I'm grateful for the family God placed me in

Every week, we went to church to learn about the Lord

From Sunday school to youth programs, we learned about the Word

People's lives were the biggest lessons ever taught

The love they showed each other that never could be bought

Well, my parents taught me how to serve the Lord in every way

Mercy and compassion should be used every day

Visit sick, care for elderly, a card, a call to cheer

A smile and a hope filled prayer to dispel any fear.

I'm grateful for the family God placed me in

Mom and Dad, they loved Jesus

And they kept us far from sin

A church family that loved you no matter where you'd been

I'm grateful for the family God placed me in

So we take our kids to church now to learn about the Lord

Same old stories, songs and flannel graphs

Still teaching them the Word

Yet the greatest lessons they will learn aren't in the books at all

But are the lives lived completely in submission to His call.

Maybe your family didn't teach you what was right from wrong

How to worship Jesus or sing the little songs

We're all a part of God's family, right here in this place

From each other we can learn till we see Him face to face

So I'm grateful for the family God placed me in

For a pastor who loves Jesus, helps keep us far from sin

Those who stand close beside me, throughout the thick and thin

I'm grateful for the family God placed me in.

© 2001. Julie Hayden. All rights reserved.

JULIE HAYDEN

ABOUT THE AUTHOR

Julie Hayden is a daughter, wife and mother. She cared for her mom throughout her mother's battle with Parkinson's and dementia. She continues to meet with other "Daughters of Dementia" to support and encourage them on their journey with their moms. In addition to this book, she has written and recorded two Christian music CDs. Since 2000, she has served in ministry coordinating community prayer and worship gatherings. She lives in Northwest Indiana with her husband, Randy, and their sons, Drew and Luke.

For more info, visit www.freedomvoices.net

JULIE HAYDEN

A DAUGHTER'S DIARY

JULIE HAYDEN

A DAUGHTER'S DIARY

JULIE HAYDEN